REFLECTIVE PRACTICE AND LEARNING FROM MISTAKES IN SOCIAL WORK

Alessandro Sicora

P

First published in Great Britain in 2017 by

Policy Press
University of Bristol
1-9 Old Park Hill
Bristol BS2 8BB
UK
t: +44 (0)117 954 5940
e: pp-info@bristol.ac.uk
www.policypress.co.uk

North American office:
Policy Press
c/o The University of Chicago Press
1427 East 60th Street
Chicago, IL 60637, USA
t: +1 773 702 7700
f: +1 773-702-9756
e:sales@press.uchicago.edu
www.press.uchicago.edu

British Library Cataloguing in Publication Data
A catalogue record for this book is available from the British Library.

Library of Congress Cataloging-in-Publication Data
A catalog record for this book has been requested.

ISBN 978-1-4473-2522-2 (paperback)
ISBN 978-1-4473-2523-9 (ePub)
ISBN 978-1-4473-2524-6 (Kindle)

Cover design by Andrew Corbett
Front cover: image kindly supplied by Andrew Corbett

Printed and bound by CPI Group (UK) Ltd, Croydon, CR0 4YY

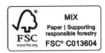

To my mother and my father

To the courageous social workers who endeavour to look at
their vulnerabilities and mistakes because they know this is the
only way to learn and also help others

Contents

List of figures and tables

Notes on the author and contributor

Alessandro Sicora is social worker and Lecturer at the University of Calabria, Italy, where he teaches Methods and Techniques of Social Work. He also teaches Theory of Social Work at the University Ca'Foscari in Venice, Italy. He has a BA in Social Work, an MA in Political Sciences and a PhD in Sociology, Social Work and Education Sciences. In the period 1990–2007 he was director of a number of small charities in Italy.

He is a Marie Curie Fellow. From 2011 to 2015 he was a member of the Executive Committee of EASSW (European Association of Schools of Social Work). Currently he is President of the Italian Society of Social Work (SocISS).

His main research interests include: methods of social work, reflexive practice, social policy. He has published books and articles on these topics.

Michael Preston-Shoot, who wrote section four of chapter three of this book, is Emeritus Professor of Social Work and Executive Dean of the Faculty of Health and Social Sciences at the University of Bedfordshire, England. He is a Fellow of the Academy of Social Sciences. He was Chair of the Joint University Council Social Work Education Committee between 2005 and 2009. He was Editor of Social Work Education between 1993 and 2006 and Managing Editor of the *European Journal of Social Work* between 2003 and 2007. He is one of the Founding Editors of the journal *Ethics and Social Welfare*. He holds a National Teaching Fellowship awarded by the Higher Education Academy, of which he is now a senior Fellow.

His publications have concentrated on law and social work practice. He has completed a longitudinal study of the outcomes of teaching law to social work students. His latest research has focused on adult safeguarding and, with Suzy Braye and David Orr, he has written major studies for the Department of Health on governance and on effective practice with adults who self-neglect. His recent books include *Making good decisions: Law for social work practice*. He was Independent Chair of Luton's Local Safeguarding Children Board and Local Safeguarding Adults Board. He is now Independent Chair of Brent Safeguarding Adults Board.

Acknowledgements

The author and publishers would like to thank the following for permission to reproduce material in this book:

- Table 4.2 (Deficit-based and strength-based questions) and Table 5.1 (From blame to appreciation) are taken from Ghaye, T. (2008) *Building the reflective healthcare organisation*, Oxford: Blackwell, pp 203 and 124, reproduced by kind permission of Wiley and Sons;
- Table 4.6 (Reflective writing using the Gibbs' reflective cycle with a limited number of words) is taken from Lia, P. (n.a.) 'Using Gibbs' Reflective Cycle', Learning Support Tutor: Disability Advisory Service: King's College London, p 5 (https://www.kcl.ac.uk/campuslife/services/disability/service/Using-Gibbs-Reflective-Cycle-in-Coursework.pdf), reproduced by kind permission of Peter Lia;
- Table 5.2 (Grid to evaluate 'How reflective is my organisation?') is taken from Ingram, R., Fenton, J., Hodson, A. and Jindal-Snape, D. (2014) *Reflective social work practice*, Basingstoke: Palgrave, p 157 reproduced by kind permission of Palgrave Macmillan.

The author is indebted to Michael Preston-Shoot and Ian Michael Robinson for their advice and comments on the drafts of this book.

Introduction

If you make a mistake and do not correct it, this is called a mistake. (Confucius)

'Seeing the world as it is not' is pretty much the definition of erring – but it is also the essence of imagination, invention, and hope. (Schulz, 2010, pp 22–3)

How to introduce a book on mistakes without making mistakes? It is a question that could block anyone. Failing to write an effective introduction has a cost (the reader could decide not to continue reading this book) but postponing day after day the writing of these lines because of an impossible search for the perfect start also has a cost (the author will never finish the book and send the manuscript to the publishing company). What to choose? It is a dilemma. Social workers have to face similar dilemmas everyday. But in their case the costs are higher, much higher, because the lives of their service users are at stake. And in many situations these are fragile lives.

'Doing no harm' is one of the overarching principles mentioned in the very recent update of the 'Global definition of social work' and related commentary (IFSW and IASSW, 2014). It is clear that nobody likes to talk about his or her own mistakes because of their negative implications for service users and the professional life of any social worker. In the publishing arena of social work books and journals reflective practice is considered, mistakes are rarely a topic, and the combination of reflective practice together with mistakes is not present at all. But if someone is reading these lines it is because he or she wants to find new ideas on how to deal with mistakes. The book is intended to help readers with tools and strategies to face daily activity in the field of social work. The main basic ideas expressed in the following pages are:

- Mistakes are an inevitable part of any human reality and also the consequence of limited resources. This is true in social work as well: if in the UK there were 20 million social workers in child protection maybe there would be no cases of abuse or maltreatment at all, but where would the salary of this group of social workers come from and who would do the other necessary jobs? Paradoxically, however, the topic of mistakes is often surrounded by taboo, because it creates unpleasant feelings in people when they have to face their limits and frailties.

- A professional error involves responsibilities for minimising the harm caused and learning how to avoid similar situations in the future. Moreover, an error can even turn into an opportunity (as the proverb says 'When life gives you lemons, make lemonade') for new discoveries and more effective interventions. So social workers need to learn from their experience and mistakes, not just for the pleasure of discovering the world in depth but because they want to do better. 'Good social workers' are capable of recognising their mistakes, and immediately 'strengthening their path', reducing any damage produced and acting more effectively in future similar situations.

- Changing slightly what Dewey (1910) wrote on experience in general, anyone can see that people do not learn from their mistakes but from their *reflection* on their mistakes. The essence of any process of reflection is made of internal dialogues that are constantly animated and nourished by *questions*. The latter become 'smart questions' when they present puzzles, leading to searches and thinking in new directions and areas, which gives an opportunity to find new solutions to unresolved problems and difficult situations. These processes may occur at a personal level or may involve another person or a multiplicity of people in groups or even in organisations.

The purpose of this book is to connect the theory of reflectivity to the practice of reflectivity, offering both a theoretical framework and a series of strategies that can be used individually or together by social workers and the other people working in the same team. At the same time, some significant *experiences* of mistakes recounted by social workers (who also describe the learning that follows from them) are provided in the text, because they can lead to a deeper understanding of the potentialities of reflective practice based on mistakes.

It is widely recognised that reflective practice is very relevant in providing better professional services. Day after day social workers face situations that are mostly unique and unrepeatable and for which solutions cannot be found in textbooks. For this reason, the development of adequate expertise through *systematic and structured reflection* is of primary importance. In fact, social work students and practitioners are often invited to stop and reflect on their experience in their field practice and their daily work. Usually, it is not easy to understand events deeply enough to transform them into meaningful facts: becoming a better practitioner, however, means that personal experience and participation should lead to new learning and skills. Sitting on a chair and recalling the events of the day is often not enough: thoughts go to the point but often jump almost randomly from one image or idea to another. A structured and more focused reflection can help one get more 'juice' and more learning from experience. Moreover, some kinds of episodes lead to better results than others. It is important to focus reflection on professional errors because, while no one wants to commit errors, when they do occur questions like "Why?" "What went wrong?" "What did I do wrong?" demand an answer. This book on how to learn from mistakes for social workers is intended to develop better practitioners and, ultimately, to provide more efficient help to people who need care.

Furthermore, sometimes social workers 'need' to take the *risk of making mistakes* because, paradoxically, in many cases trying new paths is the only way to help the service user in the long term and to learn how to reduce negative outcomes in health and social services. The metaphor of Columbus landing in America 'by mistake' while looking for a new route to India can help to develop a better comprehension of the potentialities of this kind of reflection and help social workers to find new ways to face users' complex problems. Also, both *intuition* and *rational reasoning* are needed in social work practice, but they often produce systematic errors. Reflecting on these mistakes brings a better understanding of cognitive and emotional processes, and can help social workers to improve their practice.

The book is divided into five chapters. Chapter one introduces and defines reflectivity and reflective practice within the frame of the helping professions, where they are widely considered as the basis of a skilled practitioner. The discussion on this subject is briefly presented using ideas from authors such as Schön, Dewey, Michael Polanyi, Kolb, Rogers and Habermas. This chapter describes levels and types of reflection, and explores the main connections between reflection, decision making and emotions.

Chapter two focuses on mistakes in general and then in social work. The role of heuristics, which are like automatic 'shortcuts' often occurring in the reasoning process, is considered, together with some possible answers to the question 'Who decides what is right and what is not in social work?' At the end of the chapter the particular characteristics of mistakes in social work are described, using some of the outcomes from recent research undertaken on this topic. Error is described in terms of causes (for example, lack of time, training and so on) and results (such as damage in the relationship with the user, failure of the plan, burnout and so on). Learning from a mistake is one of the effects and it may occur when some specific conditions are in place.

Chapter three considers the 'good' and 'bad' aspects of mistakes in social work. Sometimes exploring new routes is the only way to find effective solutions to the complex problems of service users. But mistakes may harm people and it is important to keep clearly in mind the dividing line between acceptable mistakes and unacceptable ones is. Codes of ethics all over the world also give social workers some guidance in this field. The last section of this chapter explores social workers' responsibilities for learning and service development in the UK context.

Chapters four and five are linked and are concerned with tools and strategies for reflection on mistakes. These include, in the first of these two chapters, how to generate appropriate questions, reflective frameworks, reflective writing, creative strategies and, in the second, assertive techniques on how to receive and how to formulate feedback when someone makes a mistake and, finally, how to recognise when organisational procedures are no longer effective and need to be changed. Chapter five also deals with organisational error-prevention systems and the so-called 'Swiss cheese model' proposed by Reason (1990), which has proved to be very useful in helping to reconstruct the sequence of events that leads to an erroneous event with the production of damage.

Overall this book:

- provides strategies and techniques all social workers can apply in their everyday work;
- offers social work students a unique source for learning more during their internship, when a certain amount of mistakes are allowed as part of the learning process needed to become a professional;
- is focused on the improvement of social work skills in the interest of service users;
- contains useful suggestions for improving the organisational climate that is often poisoned by recurrent, often vague and irrelevant criticism;
- is concerned with improving organisational learning in health and social services.

The book is targeted at social workers in health and social services and Bachelors and Masters students involved in their placements. It is intended for both teaching and practice because, even if with different intensities, the need to learn more from experience is common in students with no or only a little field practice, and practitioners with a long career behind them.

To conclude, reflection, and above all reflection on mistakes, is not only technically possible but also ethically desirable because it improves the quality of services provided by social workers. This kind of activity is fed by a permanent tension over achieving something that is impossible: that is, the total elimination of any mistakes or the attempt to reach the unreachable horizon. It is a journey that may not lead to any destination, but the ultimate goal is undoubtedly personal and professional development, the achievement of sharper eyes to look at reality in a more comprehensive way and of more expert hands to shape more effective interventions.

ONE

The never-ending cycle of reflective practice

Learning outcomes

After this chapter you will be able to:

1 have an overview of the most important ideas and authors in the literature on reflective practice;
2 define and describe reflective practice (definitions, types and levels) and some connected concepts (reflection, reflection-in-action, reflection-on-action, critical reflection and thinking, theory, practical theory, practice learning);
3 look at how in social work reflective practice is connected with decision making, emotions and creativity;
4 possess the theoretical frame for the use of the tools and strategies described in the next chapters.

Introduction

Reflective practice is an essential skill across the helping professions, but what is it? This chapter will introduce and define reflectivity and reflective practice, presenting the key ideas from leading theorists, including Schön, Dewey, Kolb, Rogers and Habermas. From different perspectives (philosophical, psychological, educational, sociological) they have given the theoretical background for understanding how human beings can learn while doing.

The so-called experience–reflection–action (ERA) cycle is examined in its three components and their mutual interactions: experience (what happens to people), reflection (all the processes enabling people to learn from these experiences) and action (undertaken because of the newly gained perspective). Reflection, as a process towards a deeper understanding and awareness, constantly feeds action and deeper focused thought towards becoming a more competent professional in the interest of the service users. Using Goodman's levels of reflection (first, description and evaluation; second, conclusions transferrable to other situations; third, acknowledgement of the wider context and influences the event under scrutiny is connected with), it is possible to lead reflection towards different depths of understanding.

Decision making is also involved in this topic, and how the human mind assesses and makes decisions, combining the contribution of intuition and reasoning, using the two-systems model of Nobel Prize winner Daniel Kahneman. These two systems process the same contents (concepts) but in two different ways described by the dichotomies fast–slow, parallel–serial, automatic–controlled, effortless–effortful and others.

In this chapter metaphors are proposed to help bring theory to life, allowing readers to understand the issue in full: in the first section, voices; in the second, cycle and iceberg; in the third, exploration by diving and walking; in the fourth, Mr Spock and Charlie Brown and; finally, in the fifth section, ghosts talking to a scared child as in the film *The Sixth Sense*.

Voices on reflectivity and reflective practice

In this section reflective practice is introduced through some of the basic ideas of the most influential authors whose works have shaped current views on this issue. Tracing the 'fathers' and 'mothers' of reflective practice as the foundation for a skilled social worker is important for many reasons. One of them is to provide direction to those who want to go on to a deeper study on this topic. The voices of, first of all, Donald Schön and then, but chronologically much earlier, John Dewey are considered essential by many scholars, as stated in the review of contemporary literature proposed by Jan Fook, Sue White and Fiona Gardner (2006). According to the latter, the lack of clear disciplinary boundaries (crossing philosophy, psychology, sociology, pedagogy and others) and the complexity of the field make it extremely difficult to conduct a literature review on reflective practice and the most important connected concepts.

Nevertheless, from the chorus of many voices, those of Michael Polanyi, Carl Rogers, David Kolb and Jürgen Habermas emerge, together with others who have developed the topic in the specific field of social work in recent publications: Gould and Baldwin (2004), Redmond (2004), Fook and Gardner (2007), Maclean (2010), Knott and Scragg (2013), Forte (2014), Ingram et al (2014) and others. The contribution of Redmond will find adequate space in the next sections and chapter, but here the most important concepts leading to the idea of reflective practice are briefly recalled and described.

The reflective practitioner of Donald Schön

The work of Donald Schön (1930–1997) is essential to understand the debate that has developed over the past 30 years on the issue of reflectivity applied to professions. His book *The reflective practitioner*, published in 1983, is probably that most quoted by scholars in this field and his legacy is still strong in health and social care as well (Kinsella, 2010).

It is as true today as it was yesterday – and especially in contexts with a high degree of uncertainty and instability – that professional activity presents a continuous challenge to fulfil functions and tasks using knowledge and skills which constantly need to be updated and rethought in a kind of a constant life-long 'maintenance'. In doing so, the ability to constantly reflect on the results achieved is indispensable.

Schön starts from the observation of a widespread crisis of confidence in professional knowledge. This means, for example, that anyone who has recently entered the world of work should soon experience how hard it is when the knowledge learned at school, college or university is found to be only a guide for professional action. Only a small proportion of cases are considered 'in the books', as most of the situations met in reality are unique and far from the descriptions provided by theory.

In fact, for social workers, doctors, nurses, lawyers, engineers and any other type of professional, the practical application of theories and techniques derived from a systematic review, preferably based on scientific criteria, would be effective only in a limited number of routine cases, which are easy to solve as they are ordinary and recurring. These professions much more frequently face situations that are difficult to fit into a predetermined scheme and that are not understandable using theoretical knowledge alone. Consequently, in these situations, applying some of the most accredited rules and procedures would give poor or no results. The need to reflect on action and learn from it comes from this preliminary observation.

According to Schön, competent practitioners are those practitioners who 'know in action' and reflect on action and in the course of action. This happens when they recognise and deal with the uniqueness of the phenomena they come into contact with, especially those that are characterised by uncertainty, instability and conflicts of values. Even so, they can manage, identify and explore new paths of action that turn out to be decisive for complex professional situations. In daily practice they formulate countless assessments for which they are seldom able to express appropriate criteria, rules and procedures. Even if they make conscious use of theories and techniques based on research, they also make extensive use of tacit knowledge and skills.

What is the key to the success of such a practitioner? It is mainly the ability to search for and find the meaning of those phenomena that are beyond the interpretative capability of 'technical rationality', that is, they are beyond a form of knowledge resulting from the application of scientific theories and techniques made using deductive procedures. The process of reflection-in-action includes the search for the meaning of these particular situations and for those 'understandings' that are implicit in their action and that the expert practitioners reveal, criticise, restructure and incorporate in their actions, which become more effective because of the knowledge built during the process of reflection. In other words, action, learning and reflection have to be conducted simultaneously. Thus the resulting cognitive activity is much broader than that normally conducted using the tools of 'technical rationality' as it involves the whole person, not just the rational part.

Among the many implications highlighted by Schön in reference to an epistemology of practice based on the idea of reflection-in-action, there is also the establishment of a different relationship between practitioner and service user (with greater attention paid to the creation of collaborative practices) and between research and practice. In this area he identifies some types of 'reflective research', which are useful to create a bridge between universities and research institutions, on the one hand, and the professional world, on the other.

John Dewey: reflection as a chain fed by troubles

The importance of John Dewey (1859–1952), who lived and wrote long before Schön, and his contribution to philosophy, psychology, education and other disciplines are widely recognised. Two of his many ideas are of great relevance for the purposes of this book: reflective thought defined as a chain, and the description of the genesis of reflective thought from a state of unrest.

A thought is everything that 'goes through our heads' and is not the direct perception of one of the senses of the thinker. This kind of mental activity is like jumping from one thought to the other. But reflection is something different and:

> involves not simply a sequence of ideas, but a consequence – consecutive ordering in such a way that each determines the next as its proper outcome, while each in turn leans back on its predecessors. The successive portions of the reflective thought grow out of one another and support one another; they do not come and go in a medley. [...] The stream or flow become a train, chain, or thread. (Dewey, 1910, pp 2–3)

In Dewey's (1910, p 6) words, 'active, persistent, and careful consideration of any belief or supposed form of knowledge in the light of the grounds that support it, and the further conclusions to which it tends, constitutes reflective thought'.

What turns a simple form of 'jumping' thinking into a 'chain or train-like' form of mental activity, that is reflective thinking? And how does this process take shape? There are two sub-processes in every reflective operation: '(a) a state of perplexity, hesitation, doubt; and (b) an act of search or investigation directed towards bringing to light further facts which serve to corroborate or to nullify the suggested belief' (Dewey, 1910, p 9). The urge to find the solution and the exit from this state of unrest is the most powerful factor guiding the entire process of reflection (Dewey, 1910, p 11). In other words, when there are problems to be solved this feeds reflection, when there are no questions to be solved there is less need for reflection. So if everything goes as expected and there are no difficulties to be overcome, there is no need to search and thinking can go back to a random form, without any specific direction.

As better described in the next chapter, unexpected mistakes (all real mistakes are unexpected, and if not they are something different, that is, an act of conscious misconduct) may lead to very fruitful reflective processes because the unrest and perplexity they produce create a strong motivation to find satisfying answers to the first and most simple question that comes to mind: why?

Abandoning what is already known and taken for granted is the precondition of any reflective thinking, which consequently:

> is always more or less troublesome because it involves overcoming the inertia that inclines one to accept suggestions at their face value; it involves willingness to endure a condition of mental unrest and disturbance. Reflective thinking, in short, means judgment suspended during further inquiry; and suspense is likely to be somewhat painful. (Dewey, 1910, p 13)

The hidden iceberg: Michael Polanyi and tacit knowledge

The metaphor of the iceberg does not come from Michael Polanyi (1891–1976) but it is inspired by his work, namely by his definition of tacit knowledge. It is not easy to fully define what this concept means. Polanyi (1966, p 4) himself says:

> we can know more than we can tell. This fact seems obvious; but it is not easy to say exactly what it means. Take an example. We know a person's face, and can recognise it among a thousand, indeed among a million. Yet we usually cannot tell how we recognise a face we know. So most of this knowledge cannot be put into words.

Later in the same work he tries to define what the relationship is between so-called objective knowledge and tacit knowledge: 'suppose that tacit thought forms an indispensable part of all knowledge, then the idea of eliminating all personal elements of knowledge would, in effect, aim at the destruction of all knowledge' (Polanyi, 1966, p 20).

In other words, tacit knowledge is what one knows but cannot express or that it would be useless to do so. A pianist or an actor risks spoiling their performance if they switch their attention continuously to their fingers or their words and gestures. Even if actors know precisely what a play is and how to act it, they need to pay attention to the totality of the whole while they are acting. That is to say that they cannot abandon the flow of what they are doing.

In social work, for example, the same fusion in perceiving sensations, emotions and knowledge may be found in face-to-face interactions and communications with service users. In addition to these interesting thoughts about the different types of awareness of the subject in the course of the action, the contribution of the theory of Polanyi on tacit knowledge may recall the concept of knowing-in-action later expressed by Schön and is particularly significant because it implies the possibility that this form of knowledge, though initially hidden, is revealed, brought to awareness, described and shared with other people. It may be said that these forms of cognitive actions feed all processes of reflectivity.

Going back to the metaphor of the iceberg representing the whole of the knowledge one has, the ice below the surface of the sea is like tacit knowledge, the visible and smaller part that has emerged above the sea is explicit and formal knowledge, and reflection processes can be seen as a means of putting on a mask and flippers to dive down to explore the iceberg below the surface of the sea.

Learning as a process of transformation of experience (David Kolb and Carl Rogers)

People learn much more from their experience than from listening in a class or reading a book or a journal article. Today this seems almost an obvious statement but, for a long time, and even in many cases today, learning has been seen as the product of an intense mental activity fed by concepts in the form of words. Starting from the works of Dewey, Lewin and Piaget, David Kolb (1939–) is someone who, more than any other author before him, brought a different view to this topic when he wrote that learning is 'the process whereby knowledge is created through the transformation of experience [and] knowledge results from the combination of grasping and transforming experience' (Kolb, 1984, p 38).

When observation, reflection, concept building and action join together in sequence, they create the essence of experiential learning. In fact, learning and knowledge are deeply connected in their natures: the first is not a set of outcomes, but consists of a process continuously creating and recreating knowledge. Learning transforms experience and the resulting knowledge is so deeply connected with the thinker that it cannot even be considered an independent entity that can be acquired or transmitted to someone else in the same exact form.

Learning as a process of transformation of experience is a concept that, before Kolb's work, seems to have been a part of the thinking of the psychologist Carl Rogers (1902–87). In his *Freedom to learn* he underlines that doing is the most important origin of learning. In his words, 'significant learning takes place when the subject matter is perceived by the student as having relevance for his own purposes' and that 'self-initiated learning which involves the whole person of the learner – feelings as well as intellect – is the most lasting and pervasive' (Rogers, 1969, pp 158–62). In other words, there are two kinds of learning: cognitive learning based on academic knowledge but not focused on learner's need and desires, and experiential learning that is directly and deeply connected with the learner's life.

Jürgen Habermas and the critical theory of society

Another milestone in building the modern perspective on the role and function of reflection comes from within sociology, where reflection is seen by some authors as the main path to disclosure and to understanding the reality behind the social veil. In particular, the German philosopher and sociologist Jürgen Habermas (1929–) is considered to be an influential thinker on current views on reflection in social work. He is one of the most authoritative theorists of the Frankfurt School and recognised the importance of dominant ideologies embedded without our being aware of them in everyday life and action. He highlighted the importance of raising consciousness of these often unjust ideologies that are hidden in language, cultural norms and social habits, and legitimate social structures and educational practices, which are accepted and thought to be 'normal' (Redmond, 2004).

Especially in *Knowledge and human interests* (1971) and *Theory of communicative action* (1984), Habermas deepened these concepts and identified three learning domains: technical, practical and emancipatory. The first two are characterised by instrumental action and 'communicative action'. The domain of emancipatory learning is related to critical reflection as a means of emancipation from the dominant ideologies. In social work, it may lead to a better understanding of oppressive power dynamics and structural sources of injustices in order to confront and challenge them.

'In simple terms, Habermas saw that [...] knowledge in the emancipatory domain led to real freedom. Freedom becomes possible because emancipatory knowledge embraces critical reflection which allows for an appreciation of those forces which control, subtly or overtly, the ability to realise full human potential' (Redmond, 2004, p 14). This idea sounds in tune with one of the core mandates expressed in the most recent 'Global definition of social work' (IFSW and IASSW, 2014):

> The development of critical consciousness through reflecting on structural sources of oppression and/or privilege, on the basis of criteria such as race, class, language, religion, gender, disability, culture and sexual orientation, and developing action strategies towards addressing structural and personal barriers are central to emancipatory practice where the goals are the empowerment and liberation of people.

Experience–reflection–action: reflective practice and associated concepts

The literature on reflection and reflective practice is becoming increasingly wide. It is possible to find quite an heterogeneous variety of definitions and reviews of these definitions, with reference to specific fields such as, for example, social work, education, nursing and other disciplines within the health and social professions (among many, see, Bulman, 2004; Fook et al, 2006; Thompson and Thompson 2008; Ruch, 2009; Bolton, 2010; Taylor, 2010; Bruce, 2013; Ingram et al, 2014 and others).

It would be difficult and useless to try to summarise everything that others, often very skilfully, have proposed with the aim of giving a clear definition of the topics mentioned earlier. Writing these pages without providing a proper working definition of one of the two main concepts of this book (the other is 'mistakes'), however, would risk making global understanding of the following pages quite difficult, and would fail in helping readers to better understand and apply the basic idea of this work: that is, that social workers can learn from their mistakes and become better practitioners if they introduce some structure and method to their reflections.

For this reason, in this section the focus in defining reflection and reflective practice is represented by their outcome in terms of action, or, more precisely, in terms of more effective actions in helping service users. These two terms are not perfectly synonymous even if they are often used as such in the literature and even more often in professional conversations. The term 'practice' recalls the implication and consequences of the acts of the reflector and these are not always implicit in the word 'reflection' that is often used to describe just the mental activity without any other meaning. In this book, these terms are sometimes used in an interchangeable way so as to underline that every reflection has some consequences in the action of the social workers and that every action is a consequence of some kind of reflection. The aim of this book is to contribute to the quality of this mutual relationship between action and reflection.

In fact, the reflective process is something in between experience and subsequent moves chosen as consequences of reflection. Jasper uses the acronym ERA to summarise this circular sequence of experience, reflection, action, and states that 'basically, reflective practice means that we learn by thinking about things that have happened to us and seeing them in a different way which enables us to take some kind of action' (Jasper, 2003, p 2). This process is built around the use of the outcome of reflection (new perspective, change in awareness and self-awareness) to improve practice and make it even more ethical (Bruce, 2013).

Furthermore, reflective practice:

- is connected to present action and is in/on action (Schön, 1987);
- leads to commitment to do something after considering both thoughts and feelings (Bulman, 2004);
- involves other people's views as well when considering events and situations (Bolton, 2010).

Developing these statements starting from the first, it might be said that the 'how' and 'when' of the link between reflection and action is of vital importance in the development of the two connected concepts of **reflection-in-action** and **reflection-on-action** developed by Schön (1987, p 26):

> We may reflect *on* action, thinking back on what we
> have done in order to discover how our knowing-
> in-action may have contributed to an unexpected
> outcome. We may do so after the fact, in tranquillity,
> or we may pause in the midst of action to make what
> Hannah Arendt (1971) calls a 'stop-and-think'. In
> either case, our reflection has no direct connection
> to present action. Alternatively, we may reflect in the
> midst of action without interrupting it. In an action-
> present – a period of time, variable with the context,
> during which we can still make a difference to the
> situation at hand – our thinking serves to reshape
> what we are doing while we are doing it. I shall say,
> in cases like this, that we reflect-in-action.

In other words, knowledge comes from carefully considering
the experience and what has been done (reflection-on-action)
so as to unveil the specific kind of knowledge that is implicit
in people's patterns of action. But there is also reflection-in-
action, when there is no interruption in the flow of reflection
mixed with action, that is, when the reflection on a certain
action is embedded in the next one. It is as if one proceeds by
'trial and error' even if this process is not random but is guided
by reflection.

In the next chapters the importance of reflection on error
will be highlighted, especially in cases when social workers
have to explore and act in difficult fields, where the amount
of information is limited to begin with (for example, refugees
and recently migrated workers) and the level of risk is high for
the people involved (for example, child protection). Second,
as will be explored later, reflection does not involve only the
'intellectual part' of mental activity but is deeply connected with
feelings and emotions. It is 'a combination of thinking, emotion
and commitment to action' (Bulman, 2004, p 4).

The reflectors are inevitably connected to their environment
and other people, as appears in the interesting definition by
Bolton (2010, p 13):

Reflection is learning and developing through examining what we think happened on any occasion, and how we think others perceived the event and us, opening our practice to scrutiny by others, and studying data and texts from the wider sphere.

Reflection is an in-depth consideration of events or situations outside of oneself: solitarily, or with critical support. The reflector attempts to work out what happened, what they thought or felt about it, why, who was involved and when, and what these others might have experienced and thought and felt about it. It is looking at whole scenarios from as many angles as possible: people, relationships, situation, place, timing, chronology, causality, connections, and so on, to make situations and people more comprehensible. This involves reviewing or reliving the experience to bring it into focus. Seemingly innocent details might prove to be key; seemingly vital details may be irrelevant.

So it is clear that different perspectives lead to new discoveries and contribute to the developing deeper understanding and new forms of action.

Finally, it is important to mention that in the study of reflective practice in the literature other important and connected concepts, like **critical reflection and thinking** are frequently found. Theory, practical theory, practice wisdom and practice learning can be part of this group, though they might seem too distant and complex.

The debate on critical reflection and critical thinking is also very rich in social work (Baldwin, 2004; Fook and Gardner, 2007; Brown and Rutter, 2008; Thompson 2010; Jones, 2013). Some of the basic questions are: What are the similarities and differences between these two concepts? Or do they even express the same idea?

Critical thinking, as defined by the National Council for Excellence in Critical Thinking (Foundation for Critical Thinking, 1987), is 'the intellectually disciplined process of actively and skilfully conceptualising, applying, analysing, synthesising, and/or evaluating information gathered from, or generated by, observation, experience, reflection, reasoning, or communication, as a guide to belief and action'. In addition it leads to the recognition of assumptions behind beliefs and actions (Brookfield, 1987).

From a different perspective, Fook and Gardner (2007) suggest that reflection is deeper than thinking and, when they summarise what critical reflection is, point out that it helps in understanding the hidden links between society and individuals. In this search, posing critical questions is an important ability in developing a habit of critical thinking and becoming a critical practitioner (Jones, 2013). Baldwin (2004) overlaps critical reflection and reflection and argues that, through reflecting critically, social workers can identify the culture (made of historical, social and political aspects) in a project team.

Does reflecting critically represent the core of reflective practice? Thompson underlines the substantial convergence between these concepts and states that 'what should be happening in critically reflecting practice is that we look carefully at the situation and seek to illuminate it by drawing on relevant parts of the professional knowledge base and integrating these into a meaningful whole that is applicable to the current practice scenario' (Thompson, 2010, p 17).

Reflection as an exploration: diving deeper or walking wider?

In the previous two sections, the main features of reflection and reflective practice have been highlighted thanks to the most authoritative voices defining these two concepts. In a context of fuzzy borders this picture helps to distinguish what reflection is and what it is not.

When talking about the contribution of Polanyi, the metaphor of the iceberg was used to describe figuratively what the whole of personal knowledge is and how it is partly tacit and partly explicit, and the idea of reflection as a kind of exploration of the hidden 'ice' was evoked. So, going back to that metaphor and imagining someone diving to see what is below the sea level (that is, what is the practitioner is unaware of), how deeply can the diver explore? Going to the meaning of the metaphor, are there different levels of reflection? Or even more than one type of?

In literature some authors (for example, Goodman, 1984; Bulman and Schutz, 2013; Fook et al, 2006; Brown and Rutter, 2008) have described some levels and others (for example, Ghaye and Ghaye, 1998; Ruch, 2009; Taylor, 2010) delineate some types of reflection and reflective practice. It seems as though in both cases the authors answer the question of 'where to explore through reflection?' and this presupposes a clear awareness of the purpose ('why explore?', that is 'why reflect?'). Maybe, if the world of experience (and of the connected knowledge) is the object of reflection, this can be seen – another image! – as a planet to be explored by diving in its ocean and walking on its land. The metaphorical diving and walking are both the representation of a search for awareness, meaning and direction for new actions.

Goodman (1984) describes three **levels of reflection**:

- reflection to attain given objectives: efficiency, effectiveness and accountability are the criteria for reflection considered as a technocratic issue;
- reflection on the relationship between principles and practice: the reflector connects theory to practice and gets ready to use the learning from past experience in other similar situations;
- reflection which, besides points 1 and 2, incorporates ethical and political concerns: justice and emancipation enter the core of the reflection process and the practitioner links everyday practice to the broader context of social structure and forces.

Adding the category 'description' and 'learning', Brown and Rutter (2008) propose the following four levels, each of which has one or more key questions:

- description: awareness of relevant aspects of the experience (what, who, when, where?);
- critical analysis: exploration of underlying assumptions (how, why?);
- evaluation: expression of a judgement (how well...?);
- learning: meaning is found and new understandings and solutions are made (what does this mean?).

A more complex description of levels comes from Mezirow (1981) who, first of all, distinguishes between consciousness and critical consciousness, that is, in this last case, becoming aware of the achieved awareness. Usually Mezirow's levels of reflection incorporate those preceding them. In the first area of consciousness there are the following levels:

* reflectivity, when someone is aware of a specific perception, thought or behaviour;
* affective reflectivity, when the awareness is on the feelings produced by the way one perceives, thinks or acts;
* discriminant reflectivity, when one assesses the efficacy of perceptions, thoughts, actions and habits of doing things, and identifies the relationship between the reflector and the specific situation;
* judgemental reflectivity, which involves making and becoming aware of value judgements about perceptions, thoughts, actions and habits in terms of their being liked or disliked.

In the second group, Mezirow includes the awareness of:

* the adequacy of the concepts used to understand or judge different situations (conceptual reflectivity);
* the recognition of the habits of judging people with haste and using too limited information (psychic reflectivity);
* the reasons for conceptual inadequacy (point 5) and the habit of precipitate judgement (point 6). These reasons are rooted in cultural or psychological assumptions which are usually taken for granted, but when brought to awareness they can lead to perspective transformation, which is a concept very close to that of emancipatory action in the works of Habermas.

These contributions from Goodman, Brown and Rutter, and Mezirow help us to see the great complexity of reflections. But when looking for typologies in literature, the fields look even more complex.

Ghaye and Ghaye (1998), Ruch (2009) and Taylor (2010) identify respectively five, four and three **types of reflection**.

They are not mutually exclusive categories and can be summarised as follows:

- descriptive (reflection on what happened), perceptive (on feelings), receptive (on views of other people), interactive (on future action) and critical (on 'broader' system) reflection (Ghaye and Ghaye, 1998);
- technical (practitioners ask themselves what and how they did something and what they would do, and how, in a similar future situation), practical (practitioners ask themselves not only "What did I do and how?" but crucially "Why?"), critical (practitioners 'examine unconscious processes that might influence how they practice' and ask themselves "Why did certain behaviours arise? Why did I respond in the way I did?") and process (in addition to the previous questions practitioners seek to 'challenge the prevailing social, political and structural conditions that promote the interests of some and oppress others') reflection (Ruch, 2009, pp 23–4);
- technical, practical and emancipatory reflection. The first, using the scientific method, produces new empirical knowledge that improves instrumental action, that is, action implemented to reach a specific goal; the second generates interpretative knowledge that is useful in understanding the interpersonal basis of human experience; the third produces critical knowledge leading to liberation from oppressive forces in society (Taylor, 2010).

Finally, a synthesis of the various contributions mentioned in this section can be built around the two key words 'awareness' and 'action'. Awareness is of: behaviour, feelings, unconscious reasons of behaviour, views of others, values and principles, decision making. But also, before being aware of these things, the evaluation of the experience and action should be considered in term of effectiveness and/or efficiency and of general answers to the questions "How good is this?" "How well did I do this?"

Awareness leads to finding a meaning of the experience that is under the lenses of reflection. This meaning answers the question "Where does all this lead?" The discovery and/or building of a meaning are like a bridge between the two key words 'awareness' and 'action' and leads to the latter. So when the reflector becomes an actor both instrumental action and action leading to emancipation and liberation from oppressive forces in society become possible.

There are no clear cut borders to the 'regions' and 'seas' represented by this almost geographical representation (for example, the distinction between being a reflector and being an actor is just a conventional and logical one) but this, once again, is the consequence of the complexity of any reflection process. Like all maps, this one does not need to be a perfect representation of reality, but it has to orientate practitioners in the never-ending 'walk' to provide better help to the service users.

Reflection and decision making

Between the activity called reflection and the consequent action there is a kind of grey area called 'decision making'. It is not simply reflection, neither is it something happening and having an impact on outer reality yet, it is 'the selection of a course of action as a result of a deliberate process by one or more people' (Taylor, 2013, p 10) or, more concretely, that time frame and that set of transactions concerning the perception of a specific situation as problematic, the search for possible alternative lines, the choice of one of these and the approval of the next move, that is, its execution (Gherardi, 1989).

Every decision is made after or during some kind of reflection and leads to the resolution of an uncertainty since it implies the adhesion of the will to a project or action that has a meaning for the agent. This section contains an overview of some of the main aspects related to the interconnections between reflection and decision making, the different types of the latter, their framing and risks, plus the influence of experience versus the mechanisation brought by bureaucracy and managerialism.

This field of study is very wide and crosses psychology, sociology and other human sciences and disciplines. Any theory that tries to describe and explain decision making is labelled as decision theory. From highly formal (game theory and probability theory, for example) to more informal (intuitive theories and, more in general, any theory dealing with subjective factors) approaches, decision theories include a wide range of studies, like studies of problem solving, choice behaviour, utility theory, game theory and the like (Reber et al, 2009).

Social workers have to make many decisions as a part and consequence of their professional responsibilities and mandates. National laws and codes of ethics highlight many of these responsibilities to service users, colleagues and the broader society. Taking no decision, especially in an emergency, is also a decision and often leads to bad consequences for service users and other people involved. Child protection is the clearest example of this. Chapter three will go more deeply into this issue but for now it is important to draw attention to the fact that many of the decisions social workers must take carry a high degree of risk. In other words they are decision-making situations 'where the outcomes are uncertain and where the benefits are sought but undesirable outcomes are possible' (Taylor, 2013, p 10). As will be better explained in the next chapter, in most of the cases these 'undesirable outcomes' are labelled as errors.

Taylor (2013) describes four possible **types of decision** in social work:

- Supporting service user decisions. Providing information and helping service users to think through the available choices are some of the main tasks of social workers in this case.
- Eligibility for services. Social workers are like 'gatekeepers' to benefits and services and have to balance criteria for eligibility, needs assessment and available resources. In times of budget cuts this kind of decision is becoming increasingly difficult and problematic.
- Safeguarding decisions. Vulnerable people, like children, older people or disabled adults, need to be protected when they are at risk of harm caused by other people or by circumstances. Decisions taken on behalf of other people are particularly ethically sensitive.
- Care-planning decisions. These also include the assessment phase as the starting point of a more global process. Balancing benefits and harms is important when planning any kind of social work intervention.

Decisions in all these four categories have to be taken with the highest degree of awareness in order for them to be **defensible** and **reasonable**. Any risk assessment is highly fallible and it is impossible not to make mistakes in this field, but it is possible to raise the level of accuracy. A decision can be defined as defensible when a responsible body of co-professionals would have made the same decision in the same circumstances (Carson, 1996). This happens when (Kemshall, 2001):

• an accredited methodology is used. This means that reasonable and reliable steps have been taken to collect and evaluate information, to assess the situation and plan the intervention;
• the decision is potentially or effectively shared with colleagues. It is recorded, taken within agency policy and procedures, and emerges from shared communication and information among the staff.

The need to give a quick response even when having limited information sometimes makes it difficult to strictly follow methodological and organisational procedures. Experience leads to knowledge and learning becoming increasingly internalised, and this leads to less conscious and more intuitive decisions. At the same time it improves the ability to identify relevant factors for the decision (Taylor, 2013).

It is common to see that sometimes, when the novice asks the expert social worker something like "Why did you do that?", the latter often has to stop and think for a while before giving an answer because of the need to recall the reasons for action that are sometimes 'hidden' in internalised mechanisms. But it is clear that 'although experience is a valuable source of knowledge, social workers who rely solely on personal experiences to inform their practice run the risk of bias' (Darragh and Taylor, 2009, p 149). As a social worker says, during an interview for a research project on professional mistakes:

> I think it is also important to listen and accept what comes from inside of you, because it exists and, moreover, you cannot deny it. But it is unthinkable to make a personalised approach because personalised

approaches must not exist in any profession. And, in fact, you have to follow the methods and theoretical model you choose. This is the only way to validate your professional action. Because, if there are 35,000 personalised approaches, there is not a profession. (translation from Sicora, 2010, p 90)

The debate on subjective and objective approaches is almost never-ending in social work. In the past, old-fashioned dichotomies and questions fed endless discussions that have never completely died out, like 'Is social work an art or a science?' or 'As a social worker, is it better to base professional activity on praxis or on theory?' The apparent contrast between evidence-based practice and a softer and more reflective approach can become less distinct when, instead of looking at the 'pointing finger', the scientific and professional social work communities look at the 'pole star', that is, the promotion of 'social change and development, social cohesion, and the empowerment and liberation of people' (IFSW and IASSW, 2014), which is highlighted in the 'Global definition of social work'.

As Taylor (2013, p 73) writes: 'the essence of evidence-based practice is not that professional expertise will be rejected in favour of some mechanistic method. Rather, evidence-based practice is about consciously identifying, understanding and using the best available relevant knowledge to inform practice decisions.' Also, reflective practice works towards more consciousness and transparency in practice, and for making visible what is hidden at first sight.

The discussion is complex but, in a nutshell, it is about how the risk of 'bad' decision making can be reduced. Several attempts to give some partial answers to this key question will appear throughout this book but here, in this section focused on reflection and decision making, it is useful to transcribe a list of questions (it may be suggested that the best outputs from reflection come from 'good' questions) thought to aid reflection on professional judgements (Taylor, 2013, p 79):

- What was my role?
- What was the goal of the decision and intervention?

- What was the issue (risk) on which I had to form a judgement?
- What information about the client family and situation was most significant in shaping my judgement?
- How did the decision appear from the perspective of client problem solving?
- What assumptions influenced my judgement?
- What alternative options were considered?
- What alternative causal explanations were considered?
- What justified the decision?
- What professional knowledge informed my judgement?
- What research or theory underpinned this knowledge?
- What additional information or knowledge would I have liked to have had?
- What emotions and challenges were there in this decision situation?
- What skills did I use?
- How could my judgement have been improved?
- What learning from this might inform my judgements in future?

Another area of strategies to explore and improve decision making is that related to the **cooperative approach** involving social workers and service users together. This includes the possibility of highlighting Schön's concept of reflective service users in social work and is in tune with the idea of service users as 'experts by experience' and with the need for clear professional boundaries.

Schön defines not only the profile of the reflective practitioner but also, even if less extensively, that of the complementary figure, the **reflective client**. If the former admits to being not the only one who has important knowledge useful in facing a professional situation, and does her/his best to be connected with the client's thoughts and feelings, the latter cooperates and is involved differently from when a 'traditional contract' frame is used. The following piece of internal dialogue between a reflective client and a traditional one proposed by Schön (1983, p 302) gives a clear picture of the difference of the two situations:

Traditional contract: I put myself into the professionals' hands and, in doing this, I gain a sense of security based on faith.

Reflective contract: I join the professional in making sense of my case, and in doing this I gain a sense of increased involvement and action.

TC: I have the comfort of being in good hands. I need only comply with his advice and all will be well.

RC: I can exercise some control over the situation. I am not wholly dependent on him; he is also dependent on information and action that only I can undertake.

TC: I am pleased to be served by the best person available.

RC: I am pleased to be able to test my judgements about his competence. I enjoy the excitement of discovery about his knowledge, about the phenomena of his practice, and about myself'.

The idea of service users as 'expert by experience' has been highlighted by McLaughlin (2009) as one of the alternative ways to think about the counterparts of the social workers. Not without attracting some controversy, it emphasises the active role of service users and, somehow, the positive contribution they can bring to decision-making processes.

Nevertheless, harm and serious consequences (for example, legal action and negative psychological effects) to professionals, service users and organisations as a consequence of the violation of boundaries have been documented for doctors, nurses, psychologists, social workers and other professionals. Critical reflection is important in facing dilemmas concerning professional boundaries, because it enables practitioners to examine relational power imbalances and develop better ethical decision making (Fronek et al, 2009).

Recognising differences and complementarities in mutual respect of distinct roles can only improve the quality of the relationship between social worker and service user, and keep it alive and dynamic for effective and reflective practice.

Perhaps one of the most helpful ways of ensuring this relationship remains just and empowering is by always recalling how fine a line it is between being a professional and being a service user. At the same time there needs to be an honest acknowledgement of professional expertise and power to ensure service user perspectives and participation does not become a hollow exercise. Qualified practitioners do have expertise that is different to the service users' 'expertise on their own lives'. Practitioners must exercise their expertise responsibly and not undervalue it or allow it to be undermined. (Ruch, 2009, p 152)

But decision making can be totally deprived of meaning by the reduction of professional discretion as a consequence of bureaucratic and managerialistic organisational cultures that reduce time and space for reflection in favour of more automatic procedures, which maybe help in doing more things, but not necessarily the right thing, that is, making an effective intervention to help service users. As a worker, interviewed for the research previously mentioned, frankly said, when describing how she works:

'Work is a little struggle, trying to fill in the papers, to proceed, to make the work seem, to ourselves and to our fellow workers, perhaps even to our superiors, in some manner carried out although sometimes I am aware of its ineffectiveness. We are efficient, perhaps, but not always effective.' (in Sicora, 2010, p 63)

The risk of a non-reflective and uncritical style of work is always around the corner when organisations create preconditions. When bureaucracy and procedures become the reason for professional action and not an instrument for it, social work loses its 'soul' and is affected by a kind of perversion of its means (money, organisation and any other resources) and ends (wellbeing and citizenship rights). Today the neoliberal approach applied to social work replaces work 'with' the service users with the mere accompanying of them in a sort of 'supermarket'. From this perspective social workers would just have to clinically present the services available and the procedures for access to them (Dominelli, 2004). In this situation the space for decision making (being a service dispenser gives no need to choose because every choice is already pre-decided as an automatic reflex) is very limited and reflection is useless because it is replaced by routine responses and thoughtless practice. Less time for reflection and supervision is the direct consequence of this state of affairs, as well as the widespread tendency towards 'typification' embedded in the agency procedures. 'This tends to reduce the relationship between practitioners and service users to routine responses based on both sides of the relationship being stuck in the rigidly fixed categories of "service supplier" and "service user"' (Dolan et al, 2006, p 18). But the reality of the situations met by social workers always subverts this typification and shows how inadequate it is.

Maybe one of the ways out of this situation is to be found when decision processes are fed not only with logic and rationality but also with emotions, intuitions and anything else from the 'other' side of being human. So if, on the one hand, being perfectly rational (almost as much as a computer) would perhaps bring people to perform exact calculations on the surrounding reality, on the other hand the limits of rationality in general and, especially, of instrumental rationality in organisations where the effects mentioned earlier are produced, cannot be left unmentioned. In fact, totally rational social workers would be ineffective since emotions and empathy are basic components of any helping relationship. Motterlini (2006a), using two characters from pop culture (an alien in *Star Trek* and a child in one of the most famous cartoon strips) describes very effectively how decision making has to be developed.

> More than Mr Spock, we tend to look like Charlie Brown. And like his, even our heads are often 'hot and stupid'. But at least there is a method in 'stupidity': the mistakes we make are pervasive, recurring and predictable. They are the result of a logic different from that of mathematics, but less

systematic, the result of an ongoing negotiation process between 'automatic' processes and 'controlled' ones, between 'affect' and 'cognition' – or, more commonly, between passion and reason – and the working of synapses of the corresponding brain areas.

Yet, as masterfully documented by Antonio Damasio, in the light of numerous cases of his patients with brain lesions in the ventromedial prefrontal region, to make a 'correct' decision knowing what should be done is not enough, but it is as if we have to 'feel' it also in our body. As if pure reason needs special assistance to implement its plans, a bit of passion helps! (translated from Motterlini, 2006b: 34)

Starting from some ideas that come from what is expressed in this quotation, the next section will try to examine closely how both cognitive and emotional activities are involved in reflection and reflective practice. In social work, but maybe in all professions, rationality and reasoning are both important and needed.

Intuition and emotions vs reasoning?

Decision making is not just a question of reasoning, just as reflection is not a mere calculation. Human beings are very different from calculating machines. Maybe at some point there will be computers able to think as humans do, but at the moment the gap is still large, very large. Even if science fiction novels and films imagine a future when what is impossible now will be possible, there is still a long way to go. But creatively imagining the future and whatever is not real is one of the activities that, together with feelings and emotions, cannot be found in machines but, for good or for bad, in men and women only. This section is focused on 'the other side' of the human mind, that is, the non-rational one, and its role in reflection and reflective practice. In this perspective, the model of the two systems developed by Kahneman (2002, 2011) is becoming popular in explaining some of the most common mechanisms at the base of everyday mental activity involving System 1 (intuition) and System 2 (reasoning). The first is one of the members of the same 'family' composed of creativity, imagery, humour, emotions and moods. The impact of all these elements on reflection is strong and has to be considered for effective reflective practice, especially in social work where empathy and other 'human' qualities have a key role.

Looking at the picture of an angry face and at the calculation '17 x 24' creates two different effects: in the first case the observer immediately and intuitively recognises the mood of the man or the woman in the picture, in the second case the same person needs some time to give a meaning to those numbers when doing the multiplication, maybe with some effort and the need of paper and pencil. This experience shows how differently intuition and reasoning work in everyday life. Similar to the first example (the angry face) people react when they drive, read words on billboards, complete the sentence "bread and...", react to someone's hostile voice, recognise that an object is closer than another one, understand easy sentences and so on. Examples of similar situations to the calculation '17 x 24' are: trying to understand the meaning of this page, comparing two washing machines in order to decide which one is better to buy, parking a car in a small space, trying to remember and identify some music already heard in the past, behaving correctly in a social situation, filling in the income tax return and so on (Kahneman, 2011).

Differences and similarities between all these situations are better explained by the so-called 'model of the two systems' developed by Daniel Kahneman, Nobel Prize winner for Economics, and based on a wide range of empirical evidence. Kahneman notes that economic operators (all the people who, for example, purchase something in a shop, but also those who produce goods or services) make many mistakes and often behave in a way that is far from rational, in contrast to the assumption of rationality at the base of much of economics as a scientific discipline. This seems common to much of human behaviour in any field. When explaining this state of things, Kahneman describes two systems that are activated in processing information: System 1 – intuition and System 2 – reasoning.

How similar and how different are these two systems? And what is their relationship with a third major system represented by perception, that is, any process of becoming aware of something through sight, hearing or any of the other senses? What are the main similarities and differences in their processes and content? How do they work and what do they use?

Table 1.1 highlights the similarities and differences between perception, intuition and reasoning in their processes and content. Perception and intuition have similar processes while reasoning is different, but when it comes to the contents involved, then intuition and reasoning are similar and it is perception that is different. For example, human beings 'intuitively' think as they see things and also have intuitions in the form of mental images. Moreover sight and intuition are fast processes. More than one thing can be perceived simultaneously. This also happens with intuition, which almost automatically allows people to do more things at the same time.

How does the reasoning work? It is slow, serial (only one thing at a time can be considered and sometimes even with some effort), controlled (concentration and no distractions are needed), requires some effort and is governed by rules, such as the rules of mathematics.

Concerning the contents, however, intuition is similar to reasoning but different from perception. While the contents of perception are given by sensory stimuli (that is, perceptions in the present time), intuition also works with other objects. Perception is limited in its content to the stimulus, whereas intuition and reasoning have the same contents: the concepts. Because they process the symbols of language, intuition and reasoning can cross past, present and future.

As Kahneman (2002, p 451) explains 'the perceptual system and the intuitive operations of System 1 generate impressions of the attributes of objects of perception and thought. These impressions are not voluntary and need not be verbally explicit. In contrast, judgments are always explicit and intentional, whether or not they are overtly expressed'. Table 1.1 summarises the main characteristics, both in terms of processes and content, of the three systems previously described.

Table 1.1: Kahneman's two-systems model (adapted from Kahneman, 2002, p 451)

	PERCEPTION	INTUITION SYSTEM 1	REASONING SYSTEM 2
PROCESS	Fast Parallel Automatic Effortless Associative Slow-learning		Slow Serial Controlled Effortful Rule-governed Flexible
CONTENT	Precepts Current stimulation Stimulus-bound	Conceptual representations Past, present and future Can be evoked by language	

Reasoning and intuition 'handle' the same kind of content but work differently and, as mentioned at the end of the last section and further explained later in this book, this creates some systematic errors in human behaviour. Knowing the hidden 'rules' producing 'wrong' actions and beliefs creates precious opportunities to prevent and correct human errors in any field, including health and social services.

The process features on the left side of Table 1.1 also describe a great part of the way creativity and imagery work. In fact perception and intuition share similar functioning, especially associative mechanisms and the products of the latter are often in the form of mental images.

Giving birth to something new is the core of a creative act, even if creativity is not a phenomenon that can be found inside someone but rather in the interaction between people's thoughts and their social-cultural context. Creativity brings originality and novelty and is essential for self-knowledge, which is crucial in the scientific process even if, for example, the most common opinion is that only what is inside the conventional notion of 'objectivity' makes academic and scientific writings acceptable (McIntosh, 2010).

The reflective process has to be creative and is like an exploration into a partially known world. Looking for new answers to old or new questions is the essence of reflection but logical reasoning alone is not enough because it cannot discover innovative paths leading to finding solutions to recurring problems. Every shortcut leading to new lands and findings is useful, however unusual it is.

Even jokes and **humour** may show signs of some serious reflection behind them or can stimulate it. They may help in making use of existing awareness and in creating a new one. Both reflection and humour take essence and create awareness. In fact, from different perspectives they help in seeing underpinning patterns in people's actions and, more generally, things others may miss and/or do not see at all. Second, they lead us to meet the unexpected, to expose and unmask what is unspoken and hidden. Finally, they question and criticise conventions, but allow us to face sensitive subjects without hurting; they might even help the oppressed to cope and survive in very difficult situations (Jewish jokes in Nazi concentration camps are a good and extreme example) (Stroobants, 2009).

A reflective and funny story helps in better understanding the potential of humour. A good example of this is the following episode told by a social worker during a workshop on aggression against social workers. She was in front of a service user who appeared to be on the verge of an act of physical violence against her. Without any premeditation apart from a sudden insight, the social worker simulated an illness, as if she were fainting or having a heart attack. The social worker, who was previously in a position of power or, as the Palo Alto School says, one-up (Watzlawick et al, 1967), became powerless and in need, and so fell into the so-called 'one-down' position. This new and unexpected situation totally changed the attitude of the service user, who immediately lost his aggressiveness and took care of the social worker, bringing her a glass of water and trying to get help for her from people in nearby offices. The aggressiveness was gone as it was no longer functional in the new situation characterised by a communicative relationship (who is the helper – who is the helped?) that was now totally reversed from the usual one in that context. This episode suggests that often aggressive acts are nothing but 'desperate' attempts to escape from a position perceived as one-down as a consequence of being in front of someone who is in a one-up position (Sicora, 2013).

This story is not fiction as it is a real episode that happened to the social worker who narrated it, but the way it was told during the workshop created a funny effect. Someone there said that it was as though the former aggressive service user had become the social worker of the social worker! This helped to release tension (violence in health and social services is a sensitive topic for many workers) and the unforgettable story was better than a highly scientific objective treatise in helping those present to understand the essence of violence and work to prevent it.

The tools suggested in the following chapters to improve the quality of reflection and reflective practice make abundant use of creativity and images. Some say that manipulation of mental images not only leads to creativity, but is also the 'core process in reflective learning and reflective practice' (Gould, 1996, p 64). Metaphor, together with imagery, is essential in this process as a form of 'word-based images' and because the two 'are not simply the ornament or illustration of an underlying reality, but are themselves constitutive of knowledge' (Gould, 1996, pp 64–5). Moreover they 'function like "schemata", through which processes of accommodation and assimilation contribute, through experiential learning, to the formation of professional self-identity' (Gould, 1996, p 68) and 'underpin' 'reasoning and imagination and how we think and conceptualise our experiences' (McIntosh, 2010, p 115). In other words, metaphors are not just an ornamental part of mental processes but make an essential contribution to the exploration and understanding of the world. They deeply shape any process of selection, interconnection and building of a global and meaningful picture, starting from the different moments of daily experience

The mental manipulation of images is a central process of learning and reflective practice because, among other things, **images and metaphors** convey a holistic knowledge of action and are able to repair the breach between objectivity and subjectivity, between facts and values. This is well illustrated by Gould (1996), when he reported the description of a social work student who defined himself in field practice as an android, half man and half robot. Using this metaphor, this trainee was able to express a great variety of things that would require many words for them to be described in detail: formal theories on organisation or from sociology of the professions, feelings of alienation and of ethical dilemmas produced by the clash between aseptic bureaucratic procedures and values of respect for the individual.

Images and metaphors not only affect cognitive processes but are also strongly connected with the emotional sphere and empower reflection and reflective practice. Unfortunately, the negative side rather than the positive side of the 'non-rational' is often highlighted, which is thus seen as an obstacle rather than as a valuable ally in many professions. Even if the presence of both reason and **emotions** in every mental process is commonly accepted, the Western tradition of philosophical thinking has always considered the first far more preferable to the second. This is known as asymmetric dualism and often makes it very difficult and embarrassing for social workers to talk about their feelings (Butler, 2013).

However, the continuous exposure to the suffering of the service users inevitably involves social workers in their most intimate self because of their daily contact with the 'evil of life'. The consequent 'emotional risk' necessitates a constant attention and care, even if emotions are too often withheld, unheeded and even considered an obstacle to professionalism. Many social workers believe, or pretend to believe, that being 'professional' means they have to hold their emotions in check, to hide them and keep themselves cold and detached, protected from the interference of emotional life that threatens to 'mislead' them away from rational thoughts and behaviour. They think that this is the only way to find protection from stress and burnout.

What are emotions? What is their function? The debate raised by these two questions is really wide and it would be impossible to describe it adequately here. But when talking about reflection and reflective practice it is important to highlight that emotions alert us to the potential need to alter our goal (Butler, 2013) and help in exploring and understanding the complexity of knowledge. They 'talk' and it is always worth trying to understand their messages, even if it is not easy and some of the emotions seem inappropriate, embarrassing or scary. Sometimes people behave like the main character of the 1999 film *The sixth sense*, a child who has the gift of seeing ghosts. He is afraid of them and tries to run away because he thinks they want to hurt him. But the horror atmosphere of the story totally disappears when he understands that those dead people just want him to listen and bring their messages to their dear ones who are still alive. Stopping, listening, thinking and understanding the inner voices everybody has is an alternative but effective description of reflection.

These voices are sometimes low, sometimes loud. In this second case, in social work too, strong feelings cannot be ignored because they:

> are an indicator of ethical values. People become aroused (positively or negatively) when human values are transgressed, opposed or affirmed (examples of values are respect for my personal boundaries, trust in my professional standing, unconditional positive regard for clients [patients, students] despite race, creed or culture). Reflecting upon emotional situations can help to discover ethical values in practice. (Bolton, 2010, p 37)

Emotional self-awareness is an essential ingredient of the concept of **'emotional intelligence'**, which Daniel Goleman (1995, p 4) has popularised and defined as 'understanding one's own feelings, empathy for the feelings of others and the regulation of emotion in a way that enhances living'.

Goleman believes that emotions are an essential component in every decision-making process and are more useful when they are accepted and consciously recognised in an environment of harmony between mind and heart. Reality often confronts people with many difficult choices (How to invest money? Whom to marry?); in these cases, the learning from emotional experiences (such as a disastrous investment or a painful relationship) send signals, emotional signals, that restrict the scope of the decision by eliminating some options and highlighting others. The emotions, then, play an important role in rationality. In the complex relationship between feelings and thought, they guide decision making moment by moment, in close collaboration with the rational mind, allowing logical thinking or making it impossible. Similarly, the rational brain has a dominant role in our emotions, with the exception of those moments when people are overwhelmed by them (Goleman, 1995).

Social workers need to use the totality of themselves in their daily practice, and reflection is the proper time for building bridges between 'heart and mind'. The need to find a good balance is stated in this excerpt from one of the interviews carried out for the research on professional mistakes already mentioned:

> Intuition ends in itself; instinct can become a double-edged sword. However, if it is supported by a wealth of knowledge and experience, it can definitely be a good element for error prevention. [...] Intuition tied to my wealth of experience and experience is fine with me. Intuition controlled only by the emotional component ... I try to stop it or slow it down. (Sicora, 2010, p 91)

Reflection leads to a closer contact with emotions and in this process of discovery the first step consists in naming the emotions felt in the present or the past. Several classifications have been made to identify basic emotions and 'most would include happiness, sadness, anger, fear, surprise, anticipation and disgust. Other emotions such as envy, shame and gratitude, may be seen as stemming from or arising from various combinations of these' (Butler, 2013, p 41).

Finally, it is useful to mention that moods are similar to emotions but are less intense and last longer. They have a strong impact on thinking when reflection is upon prior experience and induces the associated mood (Sparrow, 2009). Russell (1980) created a model of emotions developed as a two-factor model: variations and combinations of pleasure and arousal generate the spectrum of moods represented in Figure 1.1.

Figure 1.1: A circumplex model of affect: direct circular scaling coordinates for 28 affect words

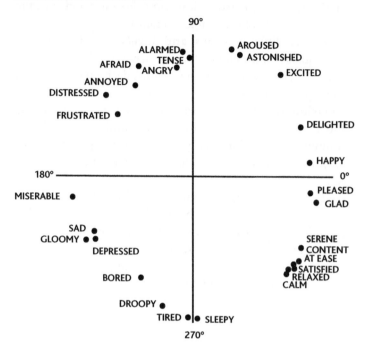

Source: Russell, 1980, p 1167

Chapter summary

1 Reflection and reflective practice are widely considered the foundation for a skilled social worker. The **debate** on this issue has been enriched by ideas from many authors (Dewey, Polanyi, Rogers, Kolb, Habermas, Schön and others). From different perspectives (philosophical, psychological, educational, sociological) their works have given the theoretical background for understanding how people can learn while doing.

2 **Reflective practice** is the result of a logical and strong connection between experience, reflection and action, which together form a never-ending cycle, bringing deeper understanding and increased effectiveness for social workers among others. The interior dialogue underlying this process is

strongly influenced and, in turn, influences the environment of the reflecting person. Searching, learning and creating theory are parts of the whole operation.

3 There are different **types and levels** of reflection as a consequence of the chosen focus (behaviours, their conscious or unconscious reasons, feelings, values, decision making) and consequent actions.

4 **Decision making** in social work needs to be defensible and reasonable (a professional methodology and shared communication with colleagues are basic requirements for this) and is improved by reflective service users and their active contribution.

5 Reflection is not only a 'rational' activity but is also deeply rooted in the 'other side' of being a human being and skilled practitioner: **imagination, creativity and emotions** bring deeper understanding and awareness of what happened, is happening and may happen, and they can provide a stronger motivation to act for the benefit of the service users.

TWO

What is a mistake in social work?

Learning outcomes

After this chapter you will be able to:

1 recognise the importance of the topic of mistakes in social work;
2 define mistakes and connected concepts in social work;
3 look at how different ideas of correctness can generate conflicts but also enrich views of social work practice and its effectiveness;
4 be aware of how intuition and heuristics may lead to mistakes;
5 possess a clear picture of the main causes and effects of mistakes in social work.

Introduction

Reflection can be carried out on any kind of experience, but reflection on mistakes is more fruitful because the unexpected failure of an action, or a series of actions, creates uneasiness in its author. These uncomfortable feelings may prompt you to look for answers to questions like "What happened? What went wrong? What did I do wrong?" in order to eliminate or reduce the discomfort that you are feeling. At the same time, reflection on mistakes is important in order to understand how to reduce the damage produced by them and to avoid repeating the same error in the future. Learning from mistakes is also ethically important on the difficult path towards the full

43

realisation of the 'doing no harm' principle that, according to the most recent 'Global definition of social work' (IFSW and IASSW, 2014), is one of the overarching principles of social work, together with respect for the inherent worth and dignity of human beings, respect for diversity, and upholding human rights and social justice.

In this chapter a **mistake** is defined as a reality of any human activity, including social work. In everyday language a mistake is an action, statement or belief that unintentionally deviates from what is correct, right or true. Then more precise and scientific definitions are given in connection to the ideas of failure and experience of error. However, *who decides what is right and what is not?* In fact it is common to find divergent answers to this basic question since a number of different subjects (social workers, service users, organisations, communities) are involved in social work interventions and might have different opinions from their particular perspective. From time to time these voices are dissonant and this leads to ethical dilemmas and conflicts, as illustrated, for example, by many situations related to child protection where the same act, such as the temporary removal of a minor from his or her family, may be considered a measure of protection or a threat to the psychological development of the child taken away from his or her original environment.

In this chapter **heuristics** and **biases** are considered together with some interesting experiments showing how some 'shortcuts' used by the human mind help in many activities but may also lead to wrong decisions. Another very useful perspective on mistakes comes from the seminal work *Human error* by James Reason (1990). He identified two main types of errors: errors in execution (I thought well, but I did wrong) and errors in planning or in problem solving (I did well, but I thought wrong). This distinction is also helpful in social work, especially when an intervention fails as a consequence of an assessment that is not in accordance with a more detailed and in-depth picture of the situation. At the end of the chapter, the particular characteristics of mistakes in social work are described, using some of the outcomes of recent research undertaken in Italy on this topic. Error is described in terms of causes (for example, lack of time, training and so on) and results (for example, damage in the relationship with the user, failure of the plan, burnout and so on). Making a mistake offers unique opportunities to learn from experience and it is important to understand the specific conditions that enable the learning process to occur.

Errors and other unpleasant events

At the centre of this and the next chapter there is an odd but very common reality: it can be called error, mistake, wrongdoing, failure or misjudgement and, among other things, it produces unpleasant feelings. Its presence in everyday life is pervasive, as is the attempt to escape from it and to deny it. This happens even if everybody knows and, from time to time, repeats old proverbs and sayings like 'never a failure, always a lesson', highlighting the importance of learning from mistakes in every aspect of existence.

Getting away from popular wisdom, error has been considered and studied by philosophers, psychologists, economists, engineers and business consultants with the purpose of limiting its likelihood and negative impact. Fallacious ideas, financial losses for corporations, mistakes in manufacturing and energy production processes, as well as in hospitals, airports and many other areas of human activity – all have been subjects of this breathless search for the paradise where there are 'zero mistakes' (Schulz, 2010). Social work is definitely one of these fields; a growing number of complaints are being raised because of the failure of professional interventions, as well as because of the pressure of public opinion, so there is a strong need to study and learn how to reduce harm sometimes caused by social workers, organisations and social policies.

'Doing no harm' is one of the overarching principles mentioned in the 'Global definition of social work' (IFSW and IASSW, 2014). And, in the same context, the complexity of the issue and the possible conflicts arising from ethical dilemmas are considered when the official 'Commentary' on that definition states: 'In some instances "doing no harm" and "respect for diversity" may represent conflicting and competing values, for example where in the name of culture the rights, including the right to life, of minority groups such as women and homosexuals, are violated' (IFSW and IASSW, 2014).

Before proposing some definitions for the topic of this chapter, it is useful to mention what Schulz (2010, p 5) calls a '**meta-mistake**', which is a mistake made when talking about mistakes. This is a wrong association of error with mere 'aberration in the normal order of things', as well as with the connected experience of embarrassment, ignorance, inattention, distraction and other reactions to the gravest social, intellectual and moral failings of human beings.

On the contrary, looking behind the meta-mistake means to discover and rediscover that the capacity to err and to reflect on errors is essential to human cognition and progress. This is the basic idea of this book even if common sense is much more focused on the negative side rather than the positive side of this concept. In fact, 'misjudgement and adverse consequences which were unplanned' is the core of the notion of mistake, according to a study involving several participants who were asked to express a definition of mistake. The scale of these consequences differentiates the latter from error and slip (Bryans, 1999, p 189). Moreover, one of the many online dictionaries defines a mistake as 'an error or fault resulting from defective judgment, deficient knowledge, or carelessness' and error as 'an act, assertion, or belief that unintentionally deviates from what is correct, right, or true' (*American Heritage® dictionary of the English language*, 2011).

On a more technical and precise level, Reason (1990, p 9) defines **error** as 'a generic term to encompass all those occasions in which a *planned sequence of mental or physical activities fails to achieve its intended outcome, and when these failures cannot be attributed to the intervention of some change agency*'. **Mistakes** are defined 'as *deficiencies or failures in the judgemental and/or inferential processes involved in the selection of an objective or in the specification of the means to achieve it, irrespective of whether or not the actions directed by this decision-scheme run according to the plan*' (Reason, 1990, p 9, emphasis in original). To these definitions that see being wrong as a deviation from an external reality, Schulz (2010, p 17) adds another, whose focus is the **experience of error**, that is the 'experience of rejecting as false a belief *we ourselves* [original emphasis] once thought was true – regardless of that belief's actual relationship to reality, or whether such a relationship can ever be determined'.

These words are important and add an interesting perspective to the topic under discussion. This seems especially useful because social reality, that is, the field where social workers are engaged day after day, is made of several and sometimes conflicting truths. What an individual or a collective considers right now could have been considered wrong in the past and vice versa. This happens not only in the controversial field of morality but also in professional fields because understanding of good practice evolves. Equally, two people can, for very good reasons and on the basis of the same information, come to two different conclusions about what is good practice in a case. For example, in medicine remedies thought efficient in the past are judged totally incorrect now. The same will probably happen for some of the treatments used at the present time to restore health. Similarly, in the same era doctors may have very different opinions on how to cure the same pathological condition.

This will also help to answer the key question 'Who decides what is right and what is wrong in social work?' in the third section of this chapter. Here and there it is also relevant to consider that the famous Thomas theorem 'If men define situations as real, they are real in their consequences' (Merton, 1948, p 193) reinforces this more complex view on error. For example, the idea that a bank will soon be unable to give money back to its account holders may be wrong, but it will become true if many people believe it is right and run to take their money back. Modern history is full of these events and in some cases only extraordinary measures taken by the authorities prevented the worst-case scenario. Many other fields of human reality provide the scene for similar phenomena, which have in common the transformation of an erroneous belief into a right one because of some particular expectations.

Going back to more stable ground and to a definition for **social work** of the first and more traditional 'external' type, Dillon (2003, pp 14–15) defines a **mistake in clinical practice** as 'an attitude, behaviour, feeling, response, communication, contextual arrangement, or strategy for work that undermines the stated purpose or specific interest of a given intervention.

Mistakes are the things we do, often unwittingly, that subvert our own conscious goals and plans with clients.'

A sequence planned to reach a desirable goal fails. Why? When this occurs because the action did not proceed as planned, there are two possible categories of error: slips (of tongue, of pen, of action), that is observable 'actions-not-as-planned', or lapses, which are more covert error forms involving failures of memory so the sequence of actions was not executed as planned (Reason, 1990, p 9).

In short, there are deviations from external reality, because the action did not proceed as planned (error in the form of a slip or lapse) or was not the right one to achieve its desired end (a mistake). Moreover, the complexity of internal changes in some beliefs that are considered no longer true constitutes the experience of error.

Close to these concepts, there are other two key words relevant to the focus of this chapter: failure and bias. Not achieving a desired end is a disturbing and sometimes even painful experience in social work. **Failures** can be met as a feeling, as a declaration from service users or as a statement from a group of workers. In this last case opinions often diverge: definitive solutions to social problems are rare and consequently it is impossible not to fail, according to some people; others think that reality is so complex that any course of action is never conclusive and can always be seen in a different light so real failures do not exist; lastly, failure always depends on expectations of the awaited results. Fronte (2008) combines these views and the possible answers to the questions like 'Does failure exist? And on what does it depend?', 'Who or what fails?' and 'How to evaluate failure' and, as summarised in Table 2.1, the outcome consists of three positions that are quite common in the social services.

The first column describes the standpoint of the 'moralist' who looks for someone (service user, social worker, the whole team) to blame. The discouraged (second column) think that the whole organisation made mistakes and that, under an innovative perspective, failures do not really exist but everything is seen as an opportunity. The last column highlights a more dialogical situation where the project of intervention and its path is considered in the light of different expectations. This generative approach is possible only if there are times and spaces when and where it is possible to combine divergent views around new hypotheses on the nature of the situations met and on how to face them. Supervision and other forms of structured reflection are of vital importance in order to have a different attitude towards failure.

Table 2.1: Three positions on failures (adapted from Fronte, 2008, p 75)

Questions/ positions	Moralist/value related	Discouraged/ innovative	Rationalist/ realist
Does failure exist? *And on what does it depend?*	It is impossible not to fail.	It does not exist.	It depends on results and expectations.
Who or what fails?	The user, the worker, the team.	The organisation.	The project or part of it.
How is failure evaluated?	Who is to blame?	Whose is the responsibility?	Where is the failure?

Biases, and most of all cognitive ones, are considered in depth in some of the most important works of Kahneman (2002, 2011). Extensive research has proved that there are systematic errors in many human intuitions that are not at all as rational as they pretend to be. Men and women go wrong when they fall into some mind traps highlighted by experimental researchers. Such errors follow some 'rules' and it is possible to be aware of them and avoid repeating the same ineffective behaviours. In fact, many errors occur because certain mental contents have a greater degree of accessibility. In other words, when some decisions have to be taken, some specific answers occur more easily, especially when there is not much time to identify the available options and choose the best one. A more thoughtful reasoning helps to identify the most correct solution.

The following is an example of these 'mind traps' (de Brabandere and Mikolajczak, 2009): if asked how many inhabitants live in Venezuela, people would give very different answers, but, if immediately before that question, someone asks them "Does Venezuela have more or less than 20 million inhabitants?", the answers will not be too far from 20 million. However, this number becomes 30 million if the question asked before is "Does Venezuela have more or less than 30 million inhabitants?"

What are these 'traps' hiding? And what will help in understanding them? Together with further examples, the next section tries to answer these questions and start to give some suggestions on how to avoid systematic errors.

Heuristics, shortcuts and errors

> Imagine that you serve on the jury of an only-child sole-custody case following a relatively messy divorce. The facts of the case are complicated by ambiguous economic, social, and emotional considerations, and you decide to base your decision entirely on the following few observations:
>
> *Parent A:* average income, average health, average working hours, reasonable rapport with the child, relatively stable social life
>
> *Parent B:* above-average income, very close relationship with the child, extremely active social life, lots of work-related travel, minor health problems. (Shafir, 1993, p 549)

This problem was presented to 170 Princeton University undergraduate volunteers. They had to choose between parent A, who has no striking positive or negative features (the words used are: average, reasonable, relatively stable), and parent B with more positive (a high income and a very close relationship with the child) and, at the same time, more negative features (health problems and lots of absences due to work-related travel).

Half of the group of volunteers had to answer to the question 'To which parent would you award sole custody of the child?' whereas the query for the other half was 'Which parent would you deny sole custody of the child?' Even if the decisions of the two groups lead to the same conclusion (if one does not receive sole custody, the other does and vice versa), the experiment has unexpected results. In fact, as shown in the following table, parent B was always chosen by the majority of the people regardless of whether the custody of the child was denied or awarded to him/her.

Table 2.2: Decisions on an only-child sole-custody case (adapted from Shafir, 1993, p 549)

	Award	Deny
Parent A	36%	45%
Parent B	64%	55%

Parent B is more likely to be chosen in both cases because he/she gives more reasons for and against being awarded sole custody of the child. It seems that it is possible to evoke the wanted answer by using the 'right' question and without the respondents being aware of what is happening.

Other similar experiments show how the framing of the instruction and other factors can heavily influence decisions on what is right and what is wrong (Kahneman, 2002). Every field of human activity is under the influence of these powerful processes leading to irrational and paradoxical decisions. How much does the form, more than the content, of communication impact on people's choices? For example, how much do reports by social workers produce 'wrong' or 'right' decisions in a third party (for example, a judge or another authority) who has the power to make a decision about the life of service users?

Complex problems (and social workers so often have to face these kinds of situations) render it difficult to make decisions. The majority of mankind would probably be stuck and frozen in endless calculations if rational, controlled and slow thinking were the only available resource. Fortunately, there are some shortcuts that make decisions possible in a reasonable time and this kind of mechanism is essential for everybody's life, especially in the case of an emergency. These simple procedures that help 'to find adequate though often imperfect answers to difficult questions' are called **heuristics** (Kahneman, 2011, p 103). In other words, a complex question is automatically and unconsciously replaced by a simpler one that can be answered more easily and in a shorter time.

To better understand how pervasive heuristics are it may be useful to try to solve this problem that Kahneman (2002, p 451) mentions in his Nobel Prize lecture: 'A bat and a ball cost $1.10 in total. The bat costs $1 more than the ball. How much does the ball cost?'

Which answer comes to mind first? The bat cost $1.00 and the ball $0.10? In most cases this is the given answer, but it is wrong because the price difference between something that costs $1 and something that costs 10 cents is 90 cents and not $1 (100 minus 10 is 90, not 100). The correct answer is: the bat costs $1.05 and the ball $0.05. Only in this case are the two requirements of the problem met: (a) $1.05 - 0.05 = 100$; (b) $1.05 + 0.05 = 1.10$.

Why is a wrong answer given more often? The need to reply fast (or the fact that it is thought that there is no need to use more time) activates a kind of 'automatic' mechanism (heuristic) that leads to error. It is easier to give the correct answer if more time to think is spent.

But why is it so easy to fall into the 'trap'? Maybe because the correct answer is 'counterintuitive' and is not found immediately, since other mental contents are more easily accessible when answering such a question.

A second interesting problem is the following: 'In a lake, there is a patch of lily pads. Every day, the patch doubles in size. If it takes 48 days for the patch to cover the entire lake, how long would it take for the patch to cover half of the lake?' (Khaneman, 2011, p 65).

Half of the lake in half the days, that is 24? It might seem so, but the correct answer is 47 days, as in the 48th day the patch doubles and covers the missing half. It could be easier to find the right solution if the respondent imagines what would happen if time could be reversed, so redoubling becomes halving: day 48, the patch is fully covered; day 47, half of the patch is covered; day 46, one fourth (that is half of the half) of the patch is covered and so on.

If the two problems are posed one after the other, and especially if they are heard rather than read, those who have experienced the unexpected difficulties of the first problem and discovered they made a mistake have usually developed a certain mistrust and caution when facing the second problem. So they do not want to reply too fast and, consequently, this enables them, through further reflection, to identify the correct answer because the one that seems right at a first glance is discarded. In other words, intuitively most people would tend to respond in the wrong way to the problem of the lake, but since the first mistake has activated some learning processes it is much easier not to be wrong when solving the second puzzle.

According to Gigerenzer et al (1999, pp 25–6), historically there are **two different approaches to heuristics**. The first, developed before the 1970s, considers them 'useful, even indispensable cognitive processes for solving problems that cannot be handled by logic and probability theory'; the second, dominant after the 1970s, views heuristics as 'mostly dispensable cognitive processes that people often misapply to situations where logic and probability theory should be applied instead'. So it seems that, especially in recent times, one of the most important 'culprits' of many human mistakes has been identified with the way people's minds decide when they have only limited time and knowledge, something that is very often the case in real life. But this raises a dilemma on what is best: to skip some important decisions in order to avoid the risk of making mistakes or to make them with the awareness that when no choice is made the consequences may be even worse than the ones of a wrong decision?

The emergency unit of a hospital is the classic situation of when, very often, decisions must be taken without any hesitation in order to save lives. These decisions are often made successfully, thanks to that mix of intuition and expertise that good practitioners have, but medicine also offers various examples of diagnostic errors and health care mistakes. Since these kinds of occurrences are systemic and, therefore, predictable, a better knowledge of the general and personal mechanisms of decision making means it is possible to implement some corrective measures for reducing suffering and saving the lives of patients (Motterlini and Crupi, 2006).

Economics is another good example of a field where heuristics very often guide people's choices in the case of urgent decisions, sometimes leading in the 'right' direction (maximising utility from the money spent) but often not. Kahneman actually won the prestigious Nobel Prize in Economic Sciences because he was able to demonstrate that humans are quite some way from being like the so-called '*homo economicus*' who is rationally capable of maximising utility as a consumer and profit as a producer.

Social work also has to deal with the limits and opportunities of rational reasoning and intuition, especially when not enough time and information are available in emergency situations, as often happens in child care services. Doing research on this and neighbouring areas of activity by constructing and using dilemmas similar to the ones mentioned earlier would be of great interest and could improve the quality of the services provided.

The **impact of heuristics** (reducing the complexity of a situation, in order to reach a decision) **and bias** (generally a negative and irrational inclination towards someone or something, similar to prejudice) is also strong in professional decision making in social work. Synthesising various sources, Taylor (2013, p 70) identifies some heuristics relevant to social work as listed in Table 2.3.

Table 2.3: Heuristics and biases (Taylor, 2013, p 70)

Anchoring bias	We often judge new situations in relation to some known 'related' point (for example, regarding normal child development or ageing) but this may be biased by an inappropriate judgement of what is normal.
Adjustment bias	Judgements may be unduly influenced by initial information that shapes our gathering and perspective on subsequent information. New information is selectively processed to support judgements already made.
Compression bias	We have a tendency to overestimate unlikely undesirable events (risk) and underestimate likely undesirable events.

Credibility bias	We may be more likely to reject something if we have a bias against the person, organisation or group to which the person belongs. We may be more inclined to accept a statement by someone we like.
Illusion of control	Humans tend to underestimate future uncertainty because we tend to believe we have more control over events than we really do.
Optimism bias	We tend to want to see things in a positive light and for them to turn out happily for all concerned.
Overconfidence	We have a tendency to be overconfident about the extent and accuracy of our personal knowledge.
Prejudice	Bias from conscious or unconscious stereotyping.
Recall bias	(similar to availability bias and recency effect) Recent and dramatic cases or incidents in the team or the media can have an undue effect. Humans have a tendency to overestimate the likelihood of types of events that are familiar from their experience or where an event of this type becomes well known through the media.
Reception bias	A willingness to believe what we have been told most often and by the greatest number of different sources.
Wariness of lurking conflict	Staff may be anxious in case they are assaulted, subject to complaints, sued, censured, criticised by inquiries, the media or politicians, and so on.

Reflective questions focused on some of the mental mechanisms described in Table 2.3 may shed more light on how decisions are taken and refine professional skills. Taylor (2013, p 72) proposed the following questions:

- What benchmarks (anchors) am I using in judging client behaviour?
- Is my practice influenced by previous experiences: (a) growing up; (b) at work; (c) adult life outside work?
- What strengths and dangers are there for professional decisions in anchoring decisions in your own previous experience?
- Am I unduly influenced by recent or dramatic events?
- What ways are there to moderate against inappropriate bias?
- How do you learn from life and work experience yet avoid bias?
- On what am I basing my estimate of the probability of harm (or success)?

- Am I giving due weight to the various sources of information?
- Am I ensuring that I do not discriminate on such grounds as sex, ethnic origin or political persuasion?
- Am I unduly confident or over-optimistic?
- What would it take to change my mind since the last assessment point?'

When reflection meets past and future experiences it becomes reflective practice and the latter cannot be done without intuition and gut feeling because they both appear quickly in consciousness and are strong enough to induce a person to act, even if there is no full awareness of the underlying reasons and processes. This happens during mental process and action. For example, when they have to kick it, football players fix their gaze on the ball, start running and adapt their speed and direction without any calculation of angles, distances and other measurements of the physical world (Gigerenzer, 2007). At the same time when social workers are dealing with an interview with a family in a difficult situation they have no time to stop, freeze the situation, go out of the room, analyse the transcript of the verbal communication and the pictures of the non-verbal communication. They have to be fully absorbed in the situation and act instantly, maybe by trial and error, so as to find appropriate questions and answers to conduct the interview.

The equilibrium between 'wrong' and 'right' intuitions is fragile and has to be found while walking a very thin line. The problem is not whether social workers need intuitions (as every human being does) but rather how they can use them and how they can transform them into evidence they can show and share.

What was said during a research project, described in the section in this chapter on 'Ethical and professional responsibilities in the UK' (p 93) by a young but already experienced worker, is enlightening:

'There are mistakes that may be of assessment in the assessment stage, the starting stage of a journey with a person, an individual project, for example [...]. But these mistakes do almost never lead to a failure, they are not the ones that determine the failure. **The ability to straighten the path according to that mistake, that is the difference.** When you skip some of the methodological passages and assess situations too superficially, do not have continuity in the project, skip the interim evaluations: this is why the project may fail, not because of a mistake of initial assessment.'

And another social worker expresses his way of creating mutual cooperation between reasoning and intuition:

'When I have to assess people in general I always start by intuition. If you ask me "do you rely completely on intuition" ... If the question is "completely?", the answer is never. But I start from listening to my intuition when it comes to assessing people. On a more detailed assessment on their personal resources it is different. It is clear. But the assessment of the people, both users and colleagues.... In the work of coordination et cetera I know that intuition can be wrong, of course. But I start from that. So I rely ... but then I always use my mind and rationality. But I think this [intuition] is a key component to be always considered in work involving relationships with people'.

Something may go wrong in every stage of the service user–social work relationship, but some initial mistakes can influence the possibility of effective interventions very negatively. According to Dillon (2003, p 96–108), some of the most frequent **mistakes in assessment** are:

- questioning without clear purpose;
- excessive focus on some things and not on others;
- lack of attention to time as structure;
- poor questioning;
- pre-empting the service user;
- not pausing for reactions to 'fact giving';

- trying to achieve too much, too soon or too little, too late;
- pressuring service users after they have balked;
- not searching out strengths if service users do not mention them;
- not being or appearing to be moved by the service user's narrative;
- not utilising multiple forms of information gathering;
- not recording information as evaluation proceeds;
- misattributing causation;
- not following up if users drop out;
- overgeneralising.

Certainly many 'to do's' and 'not to do's' might be identified for every stage of the helping process, but the complexity of the field cannot be reduced to a list of instructions whose application guarantees no mistakes are made. Sometimes instructions do not lead to the expected goals, even if they are strictly enforced, and sometimes they are unrealistic and cannot be followed, either partially or completely. The need to change strategy and explore new routes is essential for innovation and progress in every field. Thus the will to question things previously taken for granted is essential.

One of the first analyses of several inquiry reports related to mistakes in child protection work in the UK shows that the most persistent error consists of the fact that social workers are slow to revise their judgements, to accept their fallibility and to consider their assessments and consequent decisions are wrong. So information supporting one's belief is noticed much more than that which questions it (Munro, 1996).

The same conclusions are expressed in the sixth yearly national analysis of Serious Case Reviews in the UK (Brandon et al, 2012): social workers sometimes do not see what is happening in families because they fall into mental traps and find reasons to believe that even unrealistic explanations for bruises and other indicators of abuse are plausible. So they do not question themselves or others, neither do they act with stronger desire to delve beneath the appearance of events. Reflective practice and supervision are pointed out as the two most effective sources for professional improvement in child care.

Whatever it is called – overconfidence (Kahneman, 2011) or the illusion of control (Taylor, 2013) – the trap of **complacency** is always around the corner. If pilots were always overly convinced they were on the right route and, because of this unshakable certainty, never checked the on-board instrumentation, it is certain that a number of them would miss their destination or, in the worst cases, cause their airplane to crash somewhere. The ability to accept, or at least listen to alternative views from other people (for example, in this case, the co-pilot) is of vital importance even if opinion on what is right and what is wrong may differ a lot, as better described in the next section.

The changing nature of error

The metaphor of Christopher Columbus who discovered America 'by mistake' helps to better understand the changing nature of what is wrong and what is right. It is said that the Italian navigator wanted to sail to the West so as to reach India, which is to the East. He thought the Earth was a globe but smaller than it really was. With some use of the imagination, it is possible to envisage his joy when he landed on the coast after a long journey into the Atlantic Ocean in 1492. But he spent some time before realising that he was not where he wanted to be and that the people met there were not Indians. For a long time, because of this mistake, those people have been called American Indians instead of their more recent name of Native Americans. It is easy to understand the disappointment of the navigator when he understood he had not reached his destination. Who knows when that disappointment started and how long it lasted?

But at the same time it is also clear why the king and queen of Spain, who funded the Columbus expedition, were more than glad when, little by little, the opportunities from that 'mistake' emerged in terms of new land and wealth going into their hands. But what about the Native Americans? It is hard to believe they were happy to be conquered and be exterminated by the illnesses and bullets brought by Europeans. From their different perspective, Columbus has to be remembered not because he discovered America (though now it is widely recognised that it was the Vikings who first reached the American coast) but because he started the conquest of that land.

It is also interesting to mention that some time was needed to make the Europeans aware of the importance of that landing of Columbus in 1492. According to one version of what happened, Amerigo Vespucci, another explorer, but also a cartographer, was the first person who demonstrated the coast that Columbus reached was not a part of Asia but a different land (a New World, as he wrote on his maps). So cartographers after Vespucci named that new continent 'America' from his first name. Was it because Vespucci reflected more carefully on the data available on the new land on the other side the Atlantic Ocean? Maybe, but for sure only a part (Colombia), and not the entire continent, was named after Columbus.

A mistake, even a big one like the failure of Christopher Columbus to sail to India, may be considered a success or even a disaster according to the person who is evaluating it. Reflection may also transform a mistake into a success, using somebody else's enterprise, as in the case of Vespucci.

Keeping this metaphor in mind, in social work an action may be considered a mistake, a success or even a disaster, according to the person who is considering it. Any choice taken is considered correct by the worker who performs the consequent act. But what about the other people involved? What about the service users, the organisation where everything happens and what about the professional community or, in general, the 'people', public opinion or the state that defines what is right or wrong in its legislation? For example, when cases of children removed from their families because of the social workers come to the attention of the media, the differences of opinion of the subjects involved (families, social workers, managers and so on), of the social workers' community and public opinion often become very evident.

First of all, **service users** are the ones whose lives are influenced, for better or worse, by social services. It is clear that, when ethical dilemmas arise, what is beneficial for someone may be considered harmful for other people involved in the situation. In child protection services tricky situations are often part of daily practice: who and what has to be protected? The child at risk or the integrity of the family? Every social work intervention has to be an interactive and dialogic process where the voice of service users is central. It would not be in line with the principles of social work to reduce attention just to the user's point of view because service users do not have the necessary professional competence and expertise. The social worker might be right in removing a child in that by doing so he/she protects that child, but the same action can be seen as an error as it breaks up a family. The social worker might be able to justify his/her action, but for the family it could still remain an error.

Similarly, in health care, nobody who has had his/her healthy left leg amputated by mistake instead of the sick right one would consider it acceptable for the surgeon to say 'You are not competent in surgery' in reply to the complaints of the patient. Everybody would think this was an inappropriate verbal reaction because the latter, even if without any specific competence, is the one who was harmed by the wrong action. So it would be wrong to say that the patient is not qualified to judge the situation and issue a complaint, as he/she is not a surgeon.

What about the role of service users in social work? The 'Global definition of social work' highlights the importance of the involvement of service users in social work interventions as follows: 'the participatory methodology advocated in social work is reflected in "Engages people and structures to address life challenges and enhance wellbeing". As far as possible social work supports working with rather than for people' (IFSW and IASSW, 2014).

Building common expectations, understanding and planning is sometimes very difficult and may look even impossible at first sight. Child protection is the hardest field because of its complexity and the conflicting interests in play. In extreme, but not rare cases, it can even happen that social workers are attacked by service users. In fact, the very act of violent resistance is often seen as an aggression from the social workers' perspective, but as a defence from the parents' point of view, especially when they feel as if their children and their status as parents are under threat. 'Public opinion' is divided and some people think that social workers must not 'steal' children from their parents (Sicora, 2014). Involving service users and listening to their opinion on

61

what is and what is not a mistake is not only ethically important but may also make the difference between an effective and ineffective intervention. Doing things together makes it much easier to obtain the expected and agreed objectives.

The second direction from which a different voice (or, better, set of voices) on what is right or wrong may come is the **organisation**. When social workers are a part of an organisation they are subject to the opportunities and limitations arising from that collective reality. Organisations are complex systems connecting persons and things to some specific goals. So, even if from the outside they are often seen as a kind of monolith, internal conflicts are frequent because of divergent interests and views. This is also the case with mistakes. What is right for those who made the decision and acted on it may be wrong for their colleagues or according to the organisation's rules. The last chapter of this book will consider more extensively how to transform some of the problems arising from these divergences and, for example, how to use criticism (defined here as a warning received about a mistake made) as a powerful source for professional improvement, instead of an occasion of frustration. But here it is important to highlight that organisational improvement is one, even if maybe not the most common, of the possible outcomes from any dialogic debate arising from different views on what is right or wrong.

A group of friends who want to go out to have dinner together has very few, and often only implicit, rules in order to obtain their objective (that is, to spend a nice evening in each other's company). On the contrary, social services, like any other kind of organisation, need to give structure and direction to harmonise the actions of different people who often do not even know each other as people but just as functions and roles. This complex mechanism is often labelled by the term 'bureaucracy', particularly in the public sector. It is increasingly used in its negative meaning of excessive and thus inefficient regulation, rather than in its original and positive one, that of a set of regulations and structures designed to reach a specific goal. In the case of social services, this goal is wellbeing.

It often happens that, because of the complexity of organisations and their environments, procedures lose their original *raison d'*être or purpose and become in themselves the reason to do something. When filling a form becomes the goal and not the means (at the very end, the latter has always to be better services for the users), and when that specific form is no longer useful for its purpose (because it is old and social reality changes very quickly), not strictly following the procedures and not completing the form may be seen as a mistake by the organisation but not if service users are better helped by other means. Procedures are for the people, not people for the procedures. How can social workers involve themselves individually and collectively to better shape organisations when the organisations lose their original direction and mission? This is an important but very difficult question. And it is even more difficult today in the era of New Public Management or managerialism.

This may be a danger when attention is drawn to the means rather than the goal. The budget is the means not the goal. Quality certifications and other products of management decisions are 'tools' to improve life through better products and services, and when they do not do this, they have to be changed and brought back to their original purpose. As mentioned in the first chapter, the risk of a non-reflective and uncritical style of work is always around the corner when bureaucracy and procedures become the reason for professional action and not an instrument for it.

Moreover, neoliberalism is reshaping the role of the state as well as social work practice all over the world. Its emphasis on individual freedom, lack of responsibility for institutional actors, privatisation of risk and managerial administration of public sector organisations is also influencing social work.

The impact of neoliberal **managerialism** on social work can be identified in three main trends (Harris, 2014, p 16):

- *Commodification* involves identifying discrete problem categories and a menu of service options in order to quantify and cost service outputs. This often reduces social work to a series of one-off transactions, depriving it of meaningful working relationships with and commitments to service users.

- *Reducing funding to produce efficiency gains* exerts downward pressure on costs by imitating the pressure towards falling profits in capitalist markets.
- *Exerting greater control over professional space*, for example through the use of 'dashboards' as a means of heightening surveillance of the work of individual social workers and groups of social workers.

Even performance indicators may be at risk of becoming the main goal to achieve rather than the way to make visible the often invisible reality of the wellbeing of service users. If indicators do not indicate usefully they must be changed and better tools must be found. When efficiency replaces effectiveness, social workers start to look like the White Rabbit in *Alice in Wonderland*. He is always in a hurry and nobody (not even himself) really knows where he has to go, but he, enslaved by his massive watch, always has to run. What about replacing this watch with a compass to rediscover the direction of 'what really matters' in social services? Reflective practice offers the opportunity to find the lost sense of direction and restore the balance between the means and goals of social work, the techniques and values of the profession, and to find the way to change organisations when they have lost the sense of their original mission. What is 'wrong', even if according to the opinion of well qualified critics, but does work (and vice versa) has to be reconsidered in the light of the core mandates and principles of social work. What can be defined as the 'changing nature' of error makes the study of the latter especially complex and challenging.

Lastly, there is a wider and complex arena outside the relationship between service users, social workers and the organisation where the latter operate. In this space there is the **state** (any form of public authority according to the political structure of that nation) and its laws also saying what is right and what is wrong for the benefit of citizens; the **public** who, through the media express, their heterogeneous opinion; and finally the **professional and scientific communities.** These last two communities show some trends in defining what is a mistake from an ethical or a technical perspective, that is, what is bad or good in the first case, and what works and does not work in the second.

The complexity of the dynamics and diversity of the opinions makes it virtually impossible to list all the cases when something done by a social worker is considered wrong or right by different groups of people. For example, in recent years some European states (such as France and Italy) approved laws on migrants that impose actions incompatible with professional codes of conduct because of the conflicting goals of helping and controlling them. Later, in some of these cases, these regulations have been totally or partially changed, partly because of social workers' reactions. Then, what about the moving stories on TV creating outrage against social workers who take away children from their families? Are these mistakes or a mistaken way to represent events?

These pages cannot give an easy (hyper-simplified) picture of what is a mistake in social work because of the many perspectives and subjects involved. As shown by the case of Christopher Columbus, recalled at the beginning of this section, the mistake has a changing nature and has to be the source of a never-ending reflection on the basis of practice in social work, whose supreme goal is the wellbeing of service users. The questions in Table 2.4 try to propose some focus for this reflection when other people's views are considered. Then, in the next and last sections in this chapter, a type of map of causes and consequences of mistakes is drawn up according to some social workers' opinion.

Table 2.4: Different perspectives on mistakes: reflective questions

Perspective of	Reflective questions *also compare between the different perspectives arising from these questions*
Service users	• **According to your experience,** what do service users usually **expect** from social workers? What should social workers do and never do, in service users' opinion? Different people may have different expectations so can you think about different situations, different service users and related expectations? • Think about one or more **specific difficult case** you are working with **in this present time.** What are the expectations of each of the service users involved? What were their expectations at the beginning of the intervention? Now? Have they changed? How do you know what these service users expect? Did they tell you or did they express it in any other way? • In case there are divergent expectations, what can you do to **build common expectations** with service users, the whole organisation and you?
Organisation	• Are there **actions** taken by social workers for the benefit of the service users that would be **considered wrong according to the rules of your organisation**? Can you give any examples from recent situations? • Are there **rules and procedures that have lost their original functions** and no longer support the helping process for the benefit of the service users? What are the main obstacles to **changing them**? What are the factors that may contribute to changing them? What can you do to promote changing them?
Professional and scientific community	• Have you experienced **cases when you had to do something different from what is considered correct from a scientific perspective**? Have you experienced cases when you had to do something different from what is considered correct **from an ethical perspective** (for example, in contrast to the professional code of conduct)? • Can you give some examples? **Why did you act contrary to scientific evidence?** Why did you act contrary to the code of conduct?
Public opinion	• How do people see social workers? **What do people think** about what social workers would have to do and not do? Where can expressions of public opinion on this issue be seen?
Legislation	• **Which legislation may conflict with social policy** and with professional codes of ethics, and **when** and **how**? Which legislation and social policy may conflict with scientific evidence in social work, and when and how?

In the jungle of errors in social work: before, during and after

As highlighted in the previous pages, different people may consider the same action in different ways. The exploration of mistakes in social work continues in this section by listening to the voices of the workers as collected during a research project recently carried out in Italy and drawing upon some workshops and seminars on mistakes and reflective practice with hundreds of social workers in different European and non-European countries over the last decade.

In the first case, the texts collected come from the transcription of semi-structured interviews involving social workers, plus two other professions (psychologists and nurses) as a source of comparison. The questions asked relate to the perception of frequency, causes and effects of mistakes in the workplaces of the respondents, as well as self-perception on mistakes, the role of intuition and the behaviour of the respondent if a colleague is seen as making a mistake. Moreover, stories of errors have been asked for and collected.

The second source of the material used here (and, as for the research mentioned before, in the next chapters) is a series of short texts collected during training activities, as an application of a tool that will be explained in chapter four, when reflective writing will be described.

What is a mistake in social work according to the practitioners met in the circumstances above? Above all it is an event producing some kind of harm or loss of opportunity to the service user. This means, more generally, any **failure of the project of intervention** and any occurrence causing some deterioration in the relationship between social worker and user.

As a social worker says:

> 'The main effect is the failure to meet appreciable results. Social workers work to change situations. Together with their service users, they change situations, hoping to make them better. That is, they do not want to keep the existing situation unless this is the objective of the project [...]. So the bad effects

are either you do not get any change, or you get the opposite changes you had hoped for.'

Relationships are what social work practice is made up of, so it is no wonder if distrust, dissatisfaction and withdrawal from services and practitioners are considered grave consequences when something wrong has been done. This may also happen when people think they are not receiving what is their right to have from health and social services. One social worker wrote:

'A smaller, more immediate, effect is the lack of confidence in the services and public institutions. That is, basically, the change of perception of the right to welfare. In some way, the worker is a litmus test within a more complex system. Then there are perceptions of injustice, which somehow depends on the relationship developed by people with the organisation providing services. So, if it is not sufficiently motivated and explained, a decision determines feelings of distrust, of inability to receive help, even of injustice. If you think, for example of [...] the elderly [who asked] for access to services like home care. Often there are situations of denial of care, when the need and the importance of this intervention is underestimated, these situations are lived with a sense of denial of social citizenship'.

When talking about mistakes in social work, relationships are both causes and effects. Not keeping the 'right' distance, that is, when social workers behave like friends or, at the other extreme, cold and mechanical bureaucrats, is one of the most dangerous preconditions for the entire helping process to fail, as evidenced by this social worker:

'Surely some mistakes in my field are relational, that is, how you connect with people. Because as a consequence of the relationship you establish with the people, with their network et cetera, then you get the results or not. Your relational skills are very important: so consequently many errors come from unprofessionalism. Since every relationship is in our human nature, many mistakes come from the way you set the initial contact, for example, when you try to establish a kind of a friendship or a cold and distant link'.

As a very short description of a mistake of this kind and of the consequent learning, a social worker wrote two sentences, the second of which contains the learning achieved (expressed as a kind of precept): 'I started a manipulative and confidential relationship that leads to the rejection of the professional relationship. Define the right distance at the beginning of the contact!' In many cases a false step when the user meets the service for the first time may lead to even worse consequences, as can be seen in this quote: 'Poor assessment and reception by social workers caused aggression to one of them from a psychiatric patient. We must assess the situation carefully in order to avoid negative consequences.'

Listening and understanding are crucial, as this social worker's comments clearly describe: 'Difficult interview: I do not like these parents. It is useless. They do not understand. They did not listen or maybe I am the one who did not listen. Oh well, I will listen better next time' and 'Request help and orientation in a phase of acute illness. I do not listen but give just a technical reply. Humility and active and shared listening!'

Not only may the users and the professional relationship created during the intervention be harmed or damaged, but also social workers themselves are at risk of **burnout** if mistakes and failures do not find a meaning and do not become an opportunity to do better in the future, as highlighted by these comments:

> 'Another effect of the errors is the flight of the users but also the flight of the worker because there is a lot of fatigue. This is what they call burnout, isn't it? Sometimes even personal discomfort occurs because of what you have done. And you feel lonely.'

What are the **main causes** of the mistakes made in social work? The most common answers to this question from the workers met in the past years in the context described before are:

- lack of time, urgency, too much work;
- inadequate relationship with the user (as already highlighted) or with colleagues;
- inadequate organisation;
- psychological factors, such as inattention, anxiety, action without reflection, cognitive patterns that hinder a proper assessment of the situation;
- lack of training.

The most common justification when something wrong is done is the widespread conditions of **work overload** in health and social services. Too many cases and too many emergencies use up the time needed to assess more carefully, to plan more adequately and to take care of all the details needed for a successful intervention. This is summed up in one social worker's comments:

> 'So many times mistakes come from the fact that you don't have enough time to think how to do better, then you do not have time to discuss with your colleagues or to have supervision on difficult cases. We are always so pressed by the urgency of the cases and situations that we do not have a time to think what is best to do. This involves a lot of mistakes.'

Time management is often seen as a managerial obsession focused on how to improve productivity and do more with less time. As mentioned in the previous section, social workers often behave like the White Rabbit in *Alice in Wonderland*: maybe many things have been done but they are not necessarily the ones needed for a successful intervention. The ability to identify priorities and the activities that can create the strongest impact is essential, together with time to stop and reflect. It is said in the so-called Pareto principle (Kogerus and Tschäppeler, 2011) that 80% of the output is achieved with 20% of the input. But how to identity what that 20% is? Reflection and learning from the past are essential in answering this question.

It is clear that the activity of social workers is deeply connected to and influenced by the strengths and weaknesses of the organisations in which they work. Nobody, not even the person with the greatest time management ability, would be able to face hundreds of cases in the same day if forced to by his/her organisation.

> 'Poor and bad organisation.... So [many errors are] dependent not so much on the worker him/herself, but on the fact that services are organised badly for many reasons and so errors come out'.

Sometimes this happens because the regulatory framework is too rigid and unable to adapt to the real need of the people. There are conflicting powers, interests and communications. The ways of working of the individual workers are not harmonised towards service users' wellbeing. For example, as one social worker declared:

> 'The lack of internal communication in our service is a widespread problem because there is a continuous movement and even turnover of social workers and one of the most complex issues is how to share all the information [...]. We have specific tools for this, which are for example the daily meeting that brings together the whole team and allows a transfer of information between morning and afternoon shifts, a continuity in the information flow. And the shared diary, which is another tool in which the whole team cooperates in building the overall information. But, nevertheless, information is very chaotic, because the action is very fast, very chaotic, in a service like this. There are so many different things, many different levels of complexity, because we have the internal work, work with people, with groups, with their families.... There is such complexity that the information is always very complicated'.

Working collaboratively with colleagues, and not dealing with difficult situations alone, is important for social workers to be able to learn from their mistakes, as the following example demonstrates: 'Not sharing information is useless and creates tensions. Avoiding working alone and sharing ideas and projects is a tool to overcome difficulties!'

Assessment is another major area where many errors occur. It is the time when reality is mapped in order to create a plan, a series of steps to be taken for the benefit of service users. Using an inadequate map may lead to going in the wrong direction, to the failure of the helping project and even to harming some of the people involved. Some of the processes underpinning these kinds of mistake can be found in the general cognitive ones described in the second section of this chapter ('Heuristics, shortcuts and errors', p 50).

Some of the evidence given by social workers in describing their mistakes are in this area and are, for example, related to situations when some aspects are taken for granted and some information is not searched for, nor considered because the case is underestimated or considered too simple.

> 'An elderly person was found dead 20 days later because of the alarm given by neighbours. The foster person did not carry out her mandate. Being superficial in managing apparently easy cases can be risky.'

> 'I had not expected [it]. I underestimated the person, the situation. I did not expect that A would have expressed that grief. Never assume anything.'

Similarly, some areas of the life and the needs of the service user are not properly investigated: 'Fear. Psychiatric patient, homeless and jobless, wants to commit suicide. Group home available. Other services lurk. We send him there. We forgot the family dimension, the need for relationships.'

Sometimes social workers look for data confirming their first hypothesis, as in the following case: 'Alcoholic and maltreating parents with three children. Attempted but failed construction of support networks. Do not underestimate the data of reality and do not select data that only confirm the possibility of recovery.' This kind of behaviour is, of course, not limited to social workers, but extends to the generality of the people.

> Since it is rare for us to seek disruptive or nugatory evidence regarding our current beliefs for many decisions "what we see is all there is". Such a reluctance to search out broader information set can be seen to underlie three common cognitive biases:
>
> • overconfidence deriving from an inability to accept others know more,
> • framing, in accepting how information is wrapped prior to our use of it,
> • base-rate neglect, deriving from a reluctance to accept how similar we all are' (Forbes et al, 2014, p 12)

A good strategy for this kind of situation comes from the experience of another social worker who thinks it is important to have the courage to change course and writes this to describe her mistake: 'A misjudgement causes the impossibility of a post-adoptive support. For the sake of users it is good to have the courage to stop going along a route one has already started on'.

The variety of mistakes is rich in social work. Unexpected events, things forgotten, feelings unheard and overload pushing in the wrong direction are just some of the focuses of the following last short written descriptions in this chapter. Social workers wrote them as an application of the 'SMS (Short Message Service) technique', which is useful for producing extremely concise reflective writings and is described later in this book in chapter four. A specific event and the connected learning (sometimes in terms of questions for further exploration and reflection or as a sort of self-directed imperative) are described in a few words. In such cases the conciseness could reduce the clarity of the meaning:

Perhaps unexpectedly, members of family X become three. I did not reflect enough. How not to forget parts of the network and important elements in the situation?

I call a colleague to cancel an appointment and agree on further action. I do not realise immediately that the user is there. Do not treat delicate situations in overload conditions!

I am in late because I forget an appointment with a woman. She is away from her abusive husband and has two younger daughters. They are in need of help and, before the decree of the judge is issued, of some regulation for the relationship between the girls and their father.

I found out that the person who accompanied the boy to the college was not his uncle but just a friend without a strong connection with him. Maybe I had not noticed my feelings. I have to give more importance to my feelings.

There are so many opportunities to learn from mistakes and reflective practice, starting from episodes when something went wrong, is powerful in creating good practitioners. However, it is important that social workers are always fully aware that, when they make a mistake, they can always learn from it but they can also greatly damage their service users or other people involved in the situation. Balancing between these two poles (the negative and the positive implications of mistakes) is probably one of the most important skills in giving effective help, and is connected to the management of risks, responsibilities and opportunities arising in this field, as will better explained in the next chapter.

Chapter summary

1 In social work, there are deviations from external reality, because the action did not proceed as planned (this is an error in the form of a slip or a lapse) or was not the right one to achieve its desired end (this is a mistake). The complexity of internal changes in some beliefs that are considered no longer true constitutes the experience of error.

2 Intuition (and the way it generates mistakes) follows some rules when it helps in taking decisions under conditions of a shortage of time and information. It is possible to gain awareness of these rules and avoid making and/or repeating ineffective or harmful behaviour.

3 The involvement of service users in a social work intervention makes it easier to obtain the expected and agreed objectives and reduces the risks of making mistakes.

4 Social workers have to stand up and promote organisational transformation and social policy reforms when the procedures they have to follow lose their original mission of helping service users.

THREE

Risks, responsibilities and opportunities from mistakes in social work

Learning outcomes

After this chapter you will be able to:

1 be aware that errors are unpleasant but inevitable in all systems;
2 recognise the inescapable trade-off between security (and its costs) and damage caused by mistakes;
3 consider 'smart mistakes' as an alternative to failures produced by the implementation of ordinary and normal strategies;
4 gain awareness of latent errors in social work;
5 define some of the basic elements of error-prevention systems;
6 have an overview of the most important ethical and professional responsibilities for social workers in the UK and in some other countries.

Introduction

Concepts from the previous two chapters are combined in this central part of the book, which is focused on the opportunities and the risks of any learning process based on reflection on mistakes in social work. The two main questions in this context are:

- why do social workers 'need' to make mistakes or, to say it better and since everybody fails from time to time, why do they need to be more aware of their mistakes?
- what are the limits set by ethical and professional responsibilities?

The metaphor of Columbus who, as already mentioned in this book, accidentally discovered America while looking for a quicker route to India and its markets rich in spices and other precious goods, drives the explanation of the positive effects of mistakes, if (and only if) they are recognised promptly so as to minimise their negative effects and avoid repeating them in the future. Serendipity as a fortuitous discovery of something good is the basis of many important scientific innovations in medicine and other fields. It is better to be aware of mistakes and try to make the best of them since it is impossible not to make mistakes. The awareness of this simple truth may help to make the emotional experience of being wrong less unpleasant. Moreover, doing nothing just to avoid mistakes is an even bigger mistake when inaction means potential danger or harm for vulnerable people, including those who often need the help of social workers. And, if errors are inevitable, it is possible to make them 'smart', that is to use them to explore and find the way to solve problems with new solutions when the old ones do not work.

Later in this chapter special focus is given to the crucial issue of ethical and professional responsibilities. Once again the central reference point is the obligation of 'doing no harm', pointed out in the 'Global definition of social work' (IFSW and IASSW, 2014) and reinforced by some national codes of ethics (among others: the Australian Association of Social Workers, 2010; AvenirSocial, 2006; Canadian Association of Social Workers, 2005a; Consejo General de Colegios Oficiales de Diplomados en Trabajo Social y Asistentes Sociales, Espana, 1999; Danish Association of Social Workers, 2000; Deutscher Berufsverband für Soziale Arbeit, 1997; Ordine Assistenti Sociali – National Council, 2009; South African Council for Social Service Professions, 2007; Union of Social Workers, 2007), which pay attention to professional error and how to deal with it. At the same time it cannot be ignored that in many countries, when a social worker does something 'wrong', he or she might be prosecuted for the negative consequences produced. However, this is unlikely in the UK where local authorities are more likely to be held responsible for the actions of social workers unless what the social worker did or did not do is so extreme that no reasonable social worker would have done what this social worker did (Preston-Shoot, 2014). So, in order to develop a wider awareness of all the consequences of the phenomenon at the centre of the text, the main juridical implications will be described according to the current legislation in the UK.

Why do social workers 'need' mistakes?

After one of the workshops on the topic of this book in 2014, one of the participants wrote:

> 'It was a day that brought us closer to the possibility of making a mistake with less fear, the natural fear that this event brings. We were able to reflect and work on the possibility of transforming a difficult and negative event, as a mistake can be, in a new and more positive type of experience. This weakened its negative aspect and so our mistakes may appear with a more acceptable new look of "chance", "change" and "opportunity for improvement". When we deeply reflect on them, we can learn from our mistakes. If it is true that the error can cause damage, it is also true that it can become an opportunity.
>
> 'When we admit we made a mistake we do not become weaker. On the contrary, we become stronger. This requires the ability to stop and think with courage and humility. We do not need to defend ourselves, but we have to try to come closer to what is true, right, good.
>
> 'Our emotions help us in this path: when we listen to what makes us uncomfortable; with a bit of time and calmness, this discomfort may possibly find a name. We listen to ourselves, but also listen to our users, the environment, the community, the organisation where we work. This enables us to rediscover the beauty of our profession of help. These are factors that nourish and sustain our motivation: the continuous training, the feeling of belonging to

a professional community, the constant connection to our professional values.

'It is important to know ourselves, the lens that stands between us and the others, between us and what happens, the lens that we have built with our own interpretation of the facts and events.

'For this to happen, it is necessary to ensure that the reflection is not a sporadic fact [...]. It is important to know how to take space for thinking and take some distance from our frenetic activity of each day. The time to think and reflect helps us to find the compass and not to lose our way. In difficult times such as those we are living in, the ability to give priority to save a space for reflection, to know how to organise our day in order to avoid being overwhelmed by things to do, will certainly have a positive impact on ourselves and on the results of our actions.'

As the social worker who wrote those lines says, mistakes usually produce negative emotions but with courage and humility they can be transformed into an opportunity for improvement and, moreover, they can even re-motivate practitioners. To achieve these results reflection has to be a regular and systematic activity.

Starting from these thoughts this chapter is an attempt to draw a picture of the positive and negative sides of mistakes and compare them. There is such a thing as learning from mistakes but damage and harm come from the same direction. In every human field error is a powerful source of learning, it is inevitable and no-one can be fully successful in the quest for a mistake-free life in their professional activity. However, social workers have ethical ties and responsibilities towards their service users and so cannot afford to make damaging mistakes.

The two key concepts in this first section are: (1) there is no escape from a world full of mistakes, (2) it is important to do 'better failure', keeping one's eyes open for the opportunities arising from mistakes in order to balance user protection and social workers' learning. Consequently the 'need' to search for new ideas and solutions in difficult situations is highlighted, but it is important to make it clear right from the start that proceeding by 'trial and error' when the usual paths are not working has specific ethical limits and must be always conducted in the supreme interest of the service users, first of all the present ones but also those in the future, who will benefit from the actions of a more skilful practitioner.

How to find winning solutions for complex situations where the ordinary remedies are not working? The answer looks easy: by finding new ideas and methods to solve problems; but, in doing so, it is vital to be fully aware of the possible risks and to take any appropriate measure to limit them. By using the following words, attributed to Albert Einstein (Jefferson, 2016), this leads again to the core of this book: 'A person who never made a mistake never tried anything new.'

When previous attempts using ordinary and normal strategies have failed, there is little doubt that it is necessary to stray a little from the usual path. This is what Reason (1990, p 195) calls '**violations**'. These are 'deliberate – but not necessarily reprehensible – deviations from those practices deemed necessary (by designers, managers and regulatory agencies) to maintain the safe operation of a potentially hazardous system'. The same author argues that errors (mistakes, slips and lapses) are 'defined in relation to the cognitive process of the individual' but violations 'can only be described with regard to a social context in which behaviour is governed by operating procedures, codes of practice, rules and the like' (1990, p 195). Even if Reason has in mind high-technology systems, the complexity of society, human beings and their relationships makes many of the concepts developed in that context applicable in social work too. The same can be said about the principles developed by the Russian engineer Palchinsky and mentioned by Harford (2011, pp 79–80) as follows:

> What Palchinsky realised was that most real-world problems are more complex than we think. They have a human dimension, a local dimension, and are likely to change as circumstances change. His method for dealing with this could be summarised as three 'Palchinsky principles': first, seek out new ideas and try new things; second, when trying something new,

> do it on a scale where failure is survivable; third, seek out feedback and learn from your mistakes as you go along. The first principle could simply be expressed as 'variation'; the third as 'selection'. The [...] middle principle [... is] survivability [...].

In other words, the only way to find new effective ideas is first to develop and try many ideas, then to get rid of the ineffective ones after having tested them and, finally, uncovering what really works. Failure is like a tool everybody has to use in order to reach success in difficult tasks and complex situations. Only those who are ready to fail can succeed.

As mentioned in the previous chapter, the human mind often needs to use shortcuts leading to mistakes so it is important to be aware of the inevitable distortions everybody is affected by and of the irrationality in the attempt not to err at any cost (de Brabandere and Mikolajczak, 2009). In fact, sometimes the price of total security is even higher than the negative consequences of a mistake and it is very hard to balance the positive and negative outcomes of a planned action. Life has only a few ideal solutions that don't produce any kind of damage as a side effect. Best solutions are much more common but they are always 'best' for someone and not for all the people involved. **Ethical dilemmas** are common in social work and, in many situations, the borderline between what is right and what is wrong is quite controversial. What comes first: the security of a minor or the integrity of a family as the best environment for harmonious development of a child? The safety elderly people find in a retirement home or the warmth and the familiarity they have in their own houses? The autonomy of service users in their risky choices or a more or less strong pressure towards the actions considered best by the society they live in (for example, homeless people who refuse to access shelter houses)?

Freedom and mistakes are deeply linked. In this regard Mahatma Gandhi, according to many authors (Schultz, 2010, p 315), wrote that 'freedom is not worth having if it does not include the freedom to make mistakes' and an anonymous author says that 'people free to choose can make wrong choices. A world without errors would be a world without choice.' But freedom has a cost and security has a cost, too.

Reason (1990, p 203) states that:

> all organisations have to allocate resources to two distinct goals: production and safety. In the long term, these are clearly compatible goals. But, given that all resources are finite, there are likely to be many occasions on which there are short-term conflicts of interest. Resources allocated to the pursuit of production could diminish those available for safety; the converse is also true.

This bipolar dilemma 'production or safety' is aggravated in those fields where the uncertainty of the outcomes and the ambiguity of the feedback make it harder to decide which of the two poles to favour. This is true for organisations but also for individuals and in social work where there are never pure cause–effect relationships among the factors involved. For example, the security of a social worker visiting a potentially aggressive family can be enhanced by a second social worker accompanying the first one. But in doing so the second one has less time to work on other cases. Time is definitely a limited resource.

Data from the field of medicine are impressive. **Defensive medicine**, that is, when doctors order tests and treatment to avoid the risk of being prosecuted because of omissions or mistakes, has huge costs: monetary costs for the whole collective when the state pays for these precautions or health costs when, for example, exposure to unnecessary radiation may cause some pathology. In the US a recent study estimates that radiation from computed tomography could produce 1.5% to 2.0% of all cancers and 92.5% of surgeons declare they have ordered imaging tests to protect themselves from lawsuits (Hettrich et al, 2010).

This error-avoidance mindset is very common and prevents us from seeing the unexpected benefits that something wrong may bring. The following story told by a young social worker is an example of this.

'Although the error was quite trivial, it was not big, but it was an opportunity to know the person better, to discuss my mistake with him. I entered deeply into my relationship with this person by highlighting my mistake. I recognised my mistake with this person. The person has accepted it. We found a solution together and now, I must say, he and I have a great relationship and he feels somewhat more secure. It built more confidence, I believe, in us [the mental health care service team] and in me as a result of this recognition that I made explicitly. Seeing my attempt to repair my mistake, I guess, he is also better adapting to the intervention plan that he will still depend on, perhaps for a month.'

Admitting the mistake brought an even better relationship and more trust between the social worker and his service user in this case. The practitioner did not take refuge in the fortress of professional expertise and did not defend his behaviour, stressing the different roles and powers between him and his counterpart (he could have said more or less explicitly: "I know how to do things because I am a professional and I am the only one who must have power in this relationship and cannot make real mistakes.")

Analysing some error-prevention systems in health care, industry and other fields, Schulz (2010, pp 304–6) considers open and democratic communication as one of the three basic components. If a mistake is made, hiding and not admitting it is counterproductive. The other elements, deeply connected to the first one, are: the 'acceptance of likelihood of error' (whatever you do, you will always fail from time to time, so why hide it when it happens?) and 'reliance on verifiable data' (it is important to verify even small and apparently simple aspects of the planned sequence of actions in question).

The awareness of the fact that infallible error-prevention systems do not exist may lead in two opposite directions: a chronic sense of insecurity that slows activity and threatens its real effectiveness or a constant habit of investigating and keeping one's eyes wide open, not only to detect what might go wrong but also what might go unexpectedly well. The social worker mentioned earlier was able to transform a false move into a stronger relationship of trust with the user. This story may be taken as an example of **serendipity**, a concept taken up by Merton and Barber (2004) to indicate a combination of wit and luck that leads to happy and completely unintended discoveries and outcomes. Success, like failure, may come unexpectedly and even be invisible at first sight like a train that is missed if it is not seen on the platform waiting for its passengers before its departure.

Also in social work everybody needs to learn how to 'fail better' or, which is the same, make 'smart mistakes'. The 'right kind of failures' have to be 'small-scale, reversible, informative, linked to broader goals and designed to illuminate key issues' (Penn and Sastry, 2014, p 2). They have to be an exploration without doing harm. For example, social workers guide interviews with users by using disposable hypotheses and questions to go deeper into understanding situations. Verbal and non-verbal feedback from the users produces more precise conjectures that, in their turn, are verified in a continuous circular process of communication (Campanini, 2007). The workers may understand, assess and then plan only if they are absorbed in the specific situation, and enter and explore it so as to light up its more important and often hidden aspects. Inevitably, during this process, misunderstandings are possible and common but their negative consequences can be limited and turned into something positive.

How to do it? First of all, and as the 'Global definition of social work' recommends, saying that 'social work supports working with rather than for people' (IFSW and IASSW, 2014), it is important to involve service users in the process and inform them of the risks and benefits of the choices available. This principle is central in all fields but is especially important, for example, in child care. More details will follow in the third section of this chapter.

Another interesting suggestion comes from Penn and Sastry (2014) who advise people to make 'smart mistakes' going through the following three steps:

- Launch the project. It is important to plan actions but it is impossible to make them perfect because every human reality has to deal with uncertainty about the effects of action on future events. The only way to know if a project is well designed is to implement and test it.
- Build and refine through iteration. Doing is the most effective way of learning. Designing and implementing actions to generate useful insights is essential. Collecting and managing data from experimentation is also vital to make any decision system work effectively.
- Embed the learning. This can be accomplished by examining the achieved results, enhancing practice and sharing discoveries made during the whole process.

Before going on to examine the other side of the coin, that is risks and responsibilities related to mistakes in social work, it is interesting to mention some results of a qualitative and semi-structured interview based research project involving different kinds of professionals, including social workers, teachers, solicitors and human resources managers (Bryans, 1999). The analysis of the 100 interviews clearly shows that people learn more from their mistakes when they are in a safer environment and can share their learning. In every organisation managers and senior professionals have a key role in facilitating this learning, as well as initial and continuing education and training of the workers. There are also gender-related differences since women tend to internalise the blame for mistakes and men to externalise it. There is a need to enhance **'blame-free' organisational cultures**, balancing the inescapable protection of the users and the clients with maintaining the employing organisations and the individual professional's self-confidence. This, of course, does not mean to condone irresponsible organisations and practitioners but, on the contrary, to work for a more effective responsibility in enhancing the wellbeing of service users and all the other people involved in social work interventions.

The dark side of the 'planet mistake'

Everybody makes mistakes. It is such a self-evident truth that there is no need to ask people if they agree or not. But it is likely that the same people who declare their approval of this sentence would find it hard to remember and describe one or more of their mistakes. Why is there this kind of error-blindness, this strong and irresistible tendency to forget what was done wrongly (though not, of course, by others, whose mistakes are usually well remembered)?

This happens because being wrong is definitely an unpleasant experience. The awareness of the damage produced is not only negative feedback regarding professionalism but, especially for someone who has chosen a helping profession, may be felt as the failure of a wider project of life and work. So it is clear that the outcomes of a wrong action may be not only learning but also harm. The level of both can vary: the lesson learned from the experience may slip away like rain on a roof or be remembered forever so as to shape almost all future professional actions; similarly the scale of the damage may pass from irrelevant, almost non-existent, to catastrophic. This last case is rare since social workers do not have to perform open-heart surgery but wrong assessments or interventions may deeply influence people's lives. So it is important to find a way to **repair the damage produced** and draw a dividing line between where mistakes are acceptable in the search for new and more effective solutions and where it is too risky to try something new. And, most of all, in any context everybody must pay special attention to the following questions: if mistakes will always happen, what can be done to make certain that they do not damage organisations or lives irreparably?

Being wrong is an emotional experience. It is not only a recognition of a deviation from external reality and an internal change in what the subject believes and his/her consequent acts, but is also the condition 'of being stuck in real-time wrongness with no obvious way out' (Schulz, 2010, p 187). This is already **unpleasant** since nobody likes to get lost and not to know what to do (especially when you are still uncertain about what is correct), but this experience is even worse when accompanied by the sight of the damage done and when internal or external voices not only blame you for the wrong action but criticise the whole person. The shift from "I made a mistake" or "You made a mistake" to "I am a mistake" or "You are a mistake", that is "I am/you are a failure as a practitioner or even as a person" is easy and common. As explained in the last chapter, criticism may be the useful report of a mistake put forward by someone who also wants to give a constructive opportunity of learning to somebody else, but is more often done or perceived as an attack. Being to be aware of a mistake, or being forced to be aware of it, is often felt by people as sabotage to their own self-confidence and this produces more commonly a defensive reaction rather than listening and reflecting.

When the negative episode is projected over the whole personality, **shame** may be the resulting feeling. As a painful emotion due to consciousness of inadequacy, it highlights personal limits and, like any human emotion, is healthy until it is transformed into a more pervasive state.

> As a state of being, shame takes over one's whole identity. To have shame as an identity is to believe that one's being is flawed, that one is defective as a human being. Once shame is transformed into an identity, it becomes toxic and dehumanising […] and always necessitates a cover-up, a false self. (Bradshaw, 1988, pp vii–viii)

In social work this theme has recently been explored with regard to service users and how a more robust theoretical framework on shame and recognition could improve practice (Frost, 2016). But a deeper exploration with regard to social workers could be of equal interest. Shame as a state of being is hopefully rare among social workers, but many people could have experienced this feeling, even very intensely, during their career. Nevertheless, mechanisms of denial and self-defence deeply affect the quality of any intervention and may lead to the refusal to continuously work on 'maintenance' of personal work tools, like continuing training. In addition, professionalisation, when it becomes an empty fetish and a mere source of power, and some forms of organisational culture, may represent particular and largely accepted types of self-defence from the risk of a pervasive sense of inadequacy.

It is clear that in exploring the 'dark' side of mistakes, the negative consequences for service users or other people involved directly or indirectly in the intervention are definitely more important than the unpleasant emotional experiences of the social workers. Nevertheless, it is also important not to underestimate the medium- and long-term consequences of a prolonged and excessive exposure to this kind of unpleasant emotion on social workers.

There is something more to say about the connection between the good (learning and new discoveries) and the bad (harm) of mistakes. In fact, people may experience an error without damage (for example, a mathematical problem at school) or a mistake with damage (for example, in social work when a wrong assessment leads to an unnecessary separation of a child from parents). Of course, both cases are not black-and-white situations and in between there are many degrees of grey, that is, there are many intermediate levels between the two extremes of a total absence of any kind of loss and the worst catastrophe.

Then there are errors that generate learning and other similar occurrences when nothing is learned. Crossing the two dimensions 'learning' and 'damage' it is possible to build the following Figure 3.1.

Figure 3.1: Learning and damage from mistakes

Mistake	With damage	Without damage
With learning	I e.g. an unnecessary separation of a child from his/her parents	II e.g. wrong answer to a math problem
Without learning	III e.g. as above but without activation of reflective process	IV e.g. greeting a client using somebody else's name (when signs of tiredness are evident)

Source: Adapted from Sicora, 2010, p 51.

Everybody could fill this matrix with episodes from his/her professional life. The ideal situation is when the majority of them are in the II box. But this situation and the corresponding skills do not come easily and casually but are the consequence of experience and, even more, of reflecting on experience. So the purpose of this book may be visually described in Figure 3.2.

Figure 3.2: Effect of reflecting on mistakes

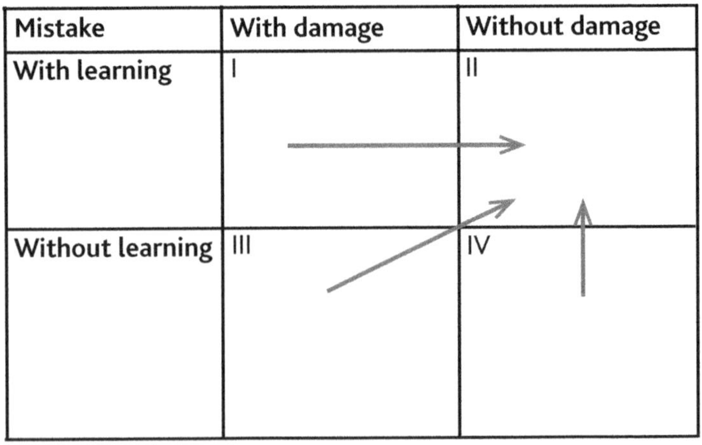

Mistake	With damage	Without damage
With learning	I	II
Without learning	III	IV

Source: Adapted from Sicora, 2010, p 51.

As said before, box II is the ideal one: always no or very little damage would be everybody's dream. But what about the opposite situation, that is, when a catastrophic event occurs? How can we learn from this major failure and prevent something similar occurring in the future?

As Reason (1990) demonstrates through the analysis of several disasters, such an event is never the consequence of a single action. On the contrary, it is always at the end of a concatenation of individually minor, but collectively catastrophic errors: of course some actions have a deeper impact than others but, nevertheless, it is useless to blame only one person and look for a scapegoat. Many of these events have been studied, especially in industry, aviation and medicine, and may teach lessons that are useful in any field of human activity (Harford, 2011, pp 217–19, emphasis added):

1. '[S]afety systems often fail'. However sophisticated they may be, prevention systems are not infallible and cannot protect against all types of risk.
2. '**[L]atent errors** can be deadly'. Reason (1990, p 173) distinguishes two kinds of error: 'active errors, whose effects are felt almost immediately, and latent errors whose adverse consequences may lie dormant within the system for a long time, only becoming evident when they combine with other factors to breach the system's defence'. Detecting latent errors is of great importance because they can lead to a disastrous outcome if combined with other factors. Paying attention to sentinel events or minor mistakes is vital in preventing catastrophic errors. Systemic or organisational changes are often required and may lead not only to averting a risk but also to general improvements in the context involved. Ignoring the existence of latent errors would be as silly as dismissing the low level of the fuel gauge and continuing to drive because you think there is no time to stop and fill the tank.
3. '[T]he third lesson is that, had whistle-blowers felt able to speak up, the accident might have been

prevented': people may be like fuel gauges in organisations when they report the existence of latent errors. The more people are free to criticise openly, the more opportunities there are to examine different points of view and discover dangerous risks or opportunities for improvement. In the last chapter of this book constructive criticism will be considered as a powerful source for transforming practitioners and organisations for the better. In this respect the expression of criticism should not be penalised but, on the contrary, rewarded.

4. '[O]ne failure tended to compound another'. When the correlation between systems is high, the effects of something that goes wrong are likely to spread more easily and worsen the final global outcome.

5. '[C]ontingency plans would have helped'. In social work these kinds of plans are often very useful, for example, in case of aggression by service users.

6. '[T]he final lesson is that of the "normal accident" theory: accidents will happen, and we must be prepared for the consequences.' The sociologist Perrow (2001, p 33), founder of this theory, argues that:

> errors are inevitable in all systems. Numerous safeguards are installed to allow correction and to limit their consequences. But in systems that have a large number of interactions that are complex, rather than linear, two or more errors, perhaps trivial in themselves, can interact in a way no designer or operator could anticipate and defeat the safeguards.

Does this mean we should surrender to the inevitability of the error? Absolutely not, this means keeping one's eyes wide open and not refusing to act just because of the fear of mistakes. Doing nothing is often worse and in many national legal systems **social workers who do not intervene** in risky situations for vulnerable people may be prosecuted, even if in the UK it is much more likely that it is an employing organisation that will be held liable for mistakes in law or in practice or both.

Social workers also fear making mistakes because they see them all as catastrophic. Sometimes this fear may lead to paralysis or to doing something, especially if some administrative procedure says so, just to show they are active and efficient, even if from the beginning it was clear that the actions performed were very likely to be ineffective in that specific situation. In social work it is important to distinguish between **'above the line'** and **'below the line'** mistakes, that is, respectively, minor and major ones. The first are an inevitable part of any intervention in a complex context. They are the 'smart mistakes' mentioned in the previous section. The second may lead to disastrous consequences. Every worker has the responsibility to know where the line is and to consider very carefully the available options, and only in extreme cases when there are no other choices take the risk after everyone who might be affected is consulted (Tugend, 2011).

Fortunately, the great majority of the mistakes social workers make are of minor importance and easily repairable and reversible. They are often recognised as infringements of methodological rules or as missing out some procedural activities. They may or may not be considered violations in the sense given by Reason (1990, p 195) to this term, as described earlier, since they are usually unwanted 'deviations from those practices deemed necessary'. Dillon (2003, pp 149–68) provides a good list of these types of errors with regard to clinical practice after the assessment phase:

- not resolving important conflicts over planning or methodology
- not helping clients obtain needed resources
- getting too far ahead of the client
- overestimating the ease of change
- skipping the middle part
- steering around topics or feelings
- not challenging or confronting the client when the process is stuck
- giving up too soon
- pushing the client
- using inappropriate or meaningless strategies

- showing favouritism
- taking sides
- defending our own points of view
- using strategies that embarrass the client
- skewing the work
- providing inadequate support and reinforcement
- scoutmaster behaviour
- 'should' and 'ought' statements
- misspeaking
- ending sessions early because the client is silent
- blaming clients for failures in the work.

Overcoming these mistakes is somehow already suggested in their description, because providing the 'not' or the 'too' is similar to showing which is the right direction to go in to repair the situation.

But it is more difficult to deal with serious mistakes and their consequences. In several countries appropriate legislation and codes of conduct have been approved to limit the risks for service users and stress the responsibility of social workers in providing professional and high-quality interventions. The remainder of this chapter focuses on these aspects of professional responsibilities.

Codes of ethics and errors in social work: a global picture

Harm, security, risk and different views on what is right and wrong are concepts related to the dark side of the 'planet mistake' as already described. Nevertheless, they are deeply connected to the ethical dimension of social work. So, in order to enrich and broaden the picture given in this chapter, an analysis of the codes of ethics in 20 countries has been undertaken to check whether and how the theme of mistakes has been considered in these codes, together with the negative consequences of mistakes (for the service users in the form of harm and for social workers in the form of sanctions from professional bodies) and the topic of criticism, that is, when social workers report mistakes to their colleagues who made them.

The countries considered are, in alphabetical order: Australia, Brazil, Canada, Denmark, France, Germany, Ireland, Israel, Italy, Japan, New Zealand, Norway, Russia, Singapore, South Africa, South Korea, Spain, Sweden, Switzerland and the US. This analysis started from the webpage of the International Federation of Social Workers (IFSW, 2016), collecting appropriate files and links and was then conducted through other internet resources provided by national professional bodies. The situation in the UK is described more extensively in the next and the last section of this chapter.

As in any other profession, the codes examined are collections of rules defining ethical practices and, as a consequence of the international status of social work, they share similar contents but also present some differences. In fact, codes of ethics are the expression of professional communities whose historical evolutions and interconnections in a global environment are complex, as may be seen through some peculiar foci found in the texts available.

In some of the countries listed, social work has a long-standing tradition, but in others it has become a recognised profession and academic discipline only recently. Consequently, the formation of a single **representative voice** for the entire professional community, as well as in relation to defining the ethical and deontological rules, is at different stages. For example, only in some nations is there a compulsory registration system managed by organisations that have become the official bodies for the profession and have been recognised by the state. The international situation is clearly not uniform and this is reflected in the presence or absence of sanctions for violation of the code (for example, the documents from France, Israel, Italy, Spain and Switzerland are very clear in defining rules for imposing penalties).

In some cases, there is explicit recognition of the value of international documents like the IFSW's 'International code of ethics' (IFSW, 2004) and/or some of the most relevant United Nations declarations on rights (the document 'Ethics in social work: an ethical code for social work professionals' by the Swedish Association of Graduates in Social Science, Personnel and Public Administration, Economics and Social Work, 2008, is one of these). In others there is acknowledgement of inspiration from other countries. For example, the Canadian Association of Social Workers (CASW) declares in its 'Code of ethics':

> The CASW also acknowledges that other codes of ethics and resources were used in the development of this Code and the Guidelines for Ethical Practice, in particular the Code of Ethics of the Australian Association of Social Workers (AASW). These resources can be found in the Reference section of each document. (2005a, p 1)

There are several terms (negligence, misconduct, misjudgement, malpractice and so on) that connote **'bad' professional behaviour** but the word 'mistake' does not appear in the documents examined. The only exception was in Russia, where social workers are invited to 'tactfully' specify service users' mistakes (Union of Social Educators and Social Workers, 2003). On the contrary, every code expresses a strong condemnation of any behaviour based on prejudice and discrimination. The term **'bias'** (used here in the second chapter to highlight the influence of cognitive processes and heuristics) is explicitly mentioned in the Australian, Israeli, South African and Russian codes.

The rest of the analysis was conducted on four main areas: (1) ethical dilemmas and conflicts of interests; (2) harm and risk; (3) reflection on practice; and (4) criticism. Even if they are all related to the responsibility of social workers to be effective practitioners guided by the overarching principle of 'doing no harm', as stated in the 'Global definition of social work' (IFSW and IASSW, 2014), the first three points are connected with the contents of the first two sections of this chapter, point 3 refers back to the content of chapter one and the last point builds a bridge to the chapter five of this book.

To begin with, **conflicts of interest** and **ethical dilemmas** are considered one of the main reasons for the existence of any code of ethics. The joint IASSW and IFSW statement and document 'International code of ethics' (2004) declares that the need to constantly reflect on challenges that face social workers and make ethically based decisions comes from the fact that social workers are both helpers and controllers, since they often have to balance the protection of service users and the social demands for efficiency and utility. Any kind of conflict of interest has to be prevented (for example, in the Israeli code) or avoided (for example, in the US) and the organisation employing social workers is often considered the main source of possible strife. In Italy, social workers must refuse to participate in any work-related activity that contradicts the code (Ordine Assistenti Sociali – National Council, 2009); in Israel 'a social worker shall undertake to receive work and to continue it only in a service whose methods of work, policy and work conditions allow him [or her] to act according to the Rules of Professional Ethics' (Union of Social Workers, 2007); and in most countries (Russia, for example) it is clearly stated that 'users come first'. Furthermore, it is interesting to note that, in order to protect social workers from often crushing organisational mechanisms, in France they cannot be considered responsible for their organisation's failure and in Italy 'a social worker must alert his [or her] employers if his [or her] work load is excessive or, if working independently, he [or she] must avoid taking on more than he [or she] can reasonably manage to achieve without prejudicing his [or her] clients' best interest' (Ordine Assistenti Sociali – National Council, 2009).

Conflicts of interests arise not only when different subjects have divergent pursuits and needs but also when different and contrasting principles lead to ethical dilemmas. These are broadly considered in the texts examined and the Swedish code deserves a mention when it stresses the toughness of assessment and declares that ethical dilemmas:

> may concern the difficulty of making priorities within a limited range of resources or of choosing the most constructive solution to a problem. Such dilemmas are often coupled to difficulties in assessing the consequences of different courses of action, e.g. the risk of a person being harmed by a measure intended to help. (Swedish Association of Graduates in Social Science, Personnel and Public Administration, Economics and Social Work, 2008, p 6)

Second, **harm and risks** are two concepts that are often mentioned to stress the role of social work as protector and defender of people and their rights. In the vast majority of the codes, the origin of harm is considered to be only outside the relationship between social workers and their service users, but in a few cases the former are explicitly asked, for example, to avoid doing any harm to the latter (Australian Association of Social Workers, 2010) or any action limiting the integrity of the user (AvenirSocial, 2006). 'Causing harm in any manner whatsoever to clients or potential clients' is listed as one of the acts that could be regarded as unethical/unprofessional behaviour in the 'Policy guidelines for course of conduct, code of ethics and the rules for social workers' of the South African Council for Social Service Professions (2007, p 40). In addition, in Italy, 'if, in carrying out his work, a social worker realises that whether by oversight or omission his client or his client's family may be harmed, he must advise the person(s) concerned accordingly and do all that he can to remedy the situation' (Ordine Assistenti Sociali – National Council, 2009, p 3).

The risk of damaging service users during an intervention is also considered in several other codes. In Australia, Germany (Deutscher Berufsverband für Soziale Arbeit, 1997), Spain (Consejo General de Colegios Oficiales de Diplomados en Trabajo Social y Asistentes Sociales, Espana, 1999) and Switzerland (AvenirSocial, 2006) social workers are clearly invited to inform users of potential risks of proposed courses of action. Similarly, Danish social workers must involve users in safe choices (Danish Association of Social Workers, 2000) and Israeli ones must 'not take responsibility for tasks where he does not have the knowledge and abilities required to execute them' (Union of Social Workers, 2007).

Interestingly, both the South African Council for Social Service Professions (2007, p 13) and the National Association of Social Workers in the US (2008) recognise the need for some forms of exploration when appropriate strategies are not available and use exactly the same words: 'when generally recognised standards do not exist with respect to an emerging area of practice, social workers should exercise careful judgment and take responsible steps (including appropriate education, research, training, consultation and supervision) to ensure competence in their work and to protect clients from harm'. Similarly, in Canada, 'social workers who engage in research minimise risks to participants, ensure informed consent, maintain confidentiality and accurately report the results of their studies' (Canadian Association of Social Workers, 2005a, p 8).

Third, **reflection** is highlighted in some codes as a precondition for ethical professional conduct. Here are some examples:

- social workers must reflect, according to the French 'Code de déontologie' approved by the Association Nationale des Assistants de Service Social (1994);
- reflection has to be 'critical' (Australian Association of Social Workers, 2010) or a 'critical self-insight' (Swedish Association of Graduates in Social Science, Personnel and Public Administration, Economics and Social Work, 2008);
- social workers have to constantly reflect on their work progress (Deutscher Berufsverband für Soziale Arbeit, 1997) or, more generally, on their activity (AvenirSocial, 2006).

Finally, reporting mistakes is sometimes considered in the form of advice, comment or **criticism**. This principle is usually stated in the section of the code on social workers' ethical responsibilities to colleagues. This is somehow connected to the general principle of accountability described in the 'International code of ethics' as: 'social workers need to acknowledge that they are accountable for their actions to the users of their services, the people they work with, their colleagues, their employers, the professional association and to the law, and that these accountabilities may conflict' (IASSW and IFSW, 2004).

As already mentioned in the first and second sections of this chapter, any error-prevention system is based on the fact that detecting latent errors is vital to prevent disastrous outcomes. If people are free or even encouraged to criticise it is easier to discover the dangers and opportunities in many situations. In the last chapter of this book this concept will be further developed alongside an attempt to identify some strategies to implement in social work services. In the codes examined, the word **'criticism'** appears more in its negative meaning, even if other terms and expressions are sometimes used to identify forms of positive feedback from colleagues or supervisors, as expressed in the following examples:

- 'social workers will relate to both social work colleagues and colleagues from other disciplines with respect, integrity and courtesy, seeking to understand differences in viewpoints and practice' (Australian Association of Social Workers, 2010, p 31);
- 'social workers remain open to constructive comment on their practice or behaviour. Social workers base criticism of colleagues' practice or behaviour on defensible arguments and concern, and deal with differences in ways that uphold the principles of the Code of Ethics, the Guidelines for Ethical Practice and the honour of the social work profession' (Canadian Association of Social Workers, 2005b, p 14);
- in New Zealand social workers have to 'remain open to constructive and informed collegial comment on professional matters and any private matter that impacts on or has the ability to impact on the social worker's service to a client or clients' (Social Workers Registration Board, Kahui Whakamana Tauwhiro, 2014, p 5);
- criticism towards colleagues must be practised in an appropriate and responsible form, according to the German code (Deutscher Berufsverband für Soziale Arbeit, 1997);
- 'social workers should seek the advice and counsel of colleagues whenever such consultation is in the best interest of the client. Consultation with a colleague would provide a perspective in terms of how a reasonable social worker would act in a particular/given situation, however, approval of the client should be sought by the practitioner before consultation' (South African Council for Social Service Professions, 2007, p 34);
- in Brazil, when social workers want to make a public criticism of a colleague, they must do so always in an objective, constructive and verifiable way, at their own risk (Conselho Federal de Serviço Social – CFESS (2011);
- in the US, the National Association of Social Workers (2008) highlights both aspects of criticism: the negative

(stating that social workers must 'avoid unwarranted negative criticism of colleagues in communications with clients or with other professionals' and 'report social work colleague's incompetence') and the positive (declaring that social workers must 'seek the advice and counsel of colleagues whenever such consultation is in the best interests of clients').

In conclusion, it is interesting to mention that some codes explicitly refer to the duty of solidarity between colleagues who should protect each other from unfair criticism. This is the case of the documents of the Japanese Association of Certified Social Workers (2004), the Union of Social Educators and Social Workers (2003) in Russia and of the South African Council for Social Service Professions ('Social workers should protect and defend colleagues against unfair criticism'; 2007, p 34). In Singapore, groundless criticism may even lead to the person being reported to the professional body, as stated in the following words: 'social workers treat with respect the professional judgment, statements and actions of colleagues. When criticisms of these appear unwarranted, social workers need to refer the matter to the Association' (Singapore Association of Social Workers, 2004).

Ethical and professional responsibilities in the UK (by Michael Preston-Shoot)

The purpose of this section is to explore social workers' responsibilities for learning and service development in one national context. If mistakes, or negative outcomes, are inevitable sometimes, even if social workers have followed the best decision-making process possible, then what approaches to analysing practice might prove fruitful in ensuring that lessons learned can be applied to future cases?

Immediately, one clarification is necessary about the UK context. Scotland and Northern Ireland have long maintained distinctive legislative systems. Wales, increasingly, is also diverging from England in the law relating to social work. Its National Assembly now has legislative competence to pass social welfare measures, akin to primary legislation (National Assembly for

Wales [Legislative Competence] [Social Welfare and Other Fields] Order 2008). Accordingly, to manage such complexity, this section will outline how legal, ethical and professional responsibilities are codified across all four nations in the UK and will distinguish where particular arrangements apply only to one specific country.

Legal standards for practice

Social workers must act lawfully when intervening in the lives of individuals and families. They must act within and not exceed their statutory authority. Thus, when seeking to safeguard children or adults from abuse or harm, social workers must appreciate how and when to exercise their responsibilities for providing care, support and protection.

Social workers must also promote **human rights** as codified in the European Convention on Human Rights, incorporated into UK law by the Human Rights Act 1998. Increasingly, too, in respect of children and young people, the different UK countries are extending the reach of the United Nations Convention on the Rights of the Child into strategic policy making but have yet to incorporate it fully into law for social work practice. Social workers must also counteract discrimination and promote equality of opportunity, as codified by the Equality Act 2010.

Administrative law lays down standards for the exercise of statutory authority. Decision making must be timely, taking account of all relevant considerations and avoiding bias. Where it is safe to do so, information must be shared and consultation take place with those involved, with reasons given for how and why particular decisions have been reached (Preston–Shoot, 2014). Practitioners and managers must act reasonably and rationally, judged against policy and legislative requirements, and prevailing social work standards. They should be mindful, therefore, of what would be expected in a particular situation of a reasonably competent social worker with professional knowledge and skills (see *Bolam* v. *Friern Hospital Management Committee* [1957]). In Scotland the similar standard is whether a social worker has acted in such a way that no similar person would have done the same if behaving with ordinary care and following normal and usual practice (*Hunter* v. *Hanley* [1955]).

One way of judging the reasonableness of decisions is to audit cases against eight literacies (Preston–Shoot, 2014), as described in Table 3.1.

Table 3.1: Key questions for auditing decisions (adapted from Preston-Shoot, 2014)

Legal literacy	Were legal options known and considered, for example on consent, safeguarding and information sharing?
Ethical literacy	Is there evidence of reflective and critical consideration and application of values, for example when balancing autonomy and a duty of care?
Professional literacy	Is there evidence that the requirements of codes of ethics and conduct were understood and applied?
Knowledge literacy	Did practitioners and managers draw on different sources of knowledge and apply these to the case?
Organisational literacy	Did social workers challenge agency and inter-agency procedures, cultures and decision making where working practices make error more likely
Relational literacy	Did social workers engage with people's biographies and lived experience, sharing concerns and perspectives with them, demonstrating curiosity, care and challenge?
Emotional literacy	How well did those involved manage stress and anxiety? Did they act with courage, resilience, integrity and respect in the face of strong emotions?
Decision-making literacy	Did practitioners and managers share information, finding time for representation, advocacy and consideration, and giving reasons for decisions?

Professional obligations

In England social workers must be registered with the Health and Care Professions Council. Standards of practice (HCPC, 2012a, 2012b) include the ability to practise lawfully, to exercise authority ethically, and to help people to stay safe, achieve and maintain independence, and feel respected and included. They must maintain public trust, for example by upholding high standards of conduct, and establishing and maintaining a safe practice environment, where concerns are raised and escalated, reasons are provided for decisions and practice is continuously reviewed. They must act within the limits of their competence and training, behave honestly and keep accurate records. They must demonstrate skills of reflection and analysis, keep their knowledge and values up to date and take responsibility for maintaining the quality of their practice. There are also knowledge and skills statements for social workers in England in adult services (DH [Department of Health], 2015a) and children's services (DfE [Department for Education], 2014), which expect social workers to understand and work effectively within relevant legal frameworks; to promote core values of human rights, equality and social justice; to be skilled in facilitating service users' participation and in taking their views into account; and to continually review and reflect upon cases as they evolve.

In Wales (Care Council for Wales, 2002, 2011), Scotland (Scottish Social Services Council, 2009, 2011) and Northern Ireland (Northern Ireland Social Care Council, 2002, 2011), the required practice standards are similarly expressed. They include being accountable for one's work, maintaining people's trust and confidence by practising professionally, and examining one's own practice. They should use evidence of what works when accounting for their decisions, be clear about their roles and responsibilities, and uphold professional ethics. They should contribute to the development of services and organisations, and provide leadership for other practitioners' learning and development. They must promote service users' engagement and participation.

The same standards for the four nations require that social workers understand the roles and responsibilities of other professionals, and are able to **work collaboratively**. These expectations are further delineated in nation-specific government guidance. For example, in England and Wales there is guidance for multi-agency working to safeguard children and young people (HM Government, 2015) and to ensure that people experiencing severe mental distress receive the care, support and protection that they need (DH, 2015b).

There are also standards for social work employers, which do not have statutory force but represent statements of good management practice. In England (LGA, 2014) the standards cover workload management, induction, continuing professional development, supervision and support, including access to legal advice, and providing a working environment where social workers can maintain their registration and escalate concerns without fear. In Wales (Care Council for Wales, 2002), Scotland (Scottish Social Services Council, 2009) and Northern Ireland (Northern Ireland Social Care Council, 2002) the standards include effective supervision and career reviews, commitment to social work values and knowledge, providing updates on law, and not jeopardising social workers' registration and licence to practise.

Reflecting on professional practice

Maintaining the quality of one's practice requires reflection. Cases can arouse strong emotions, which, if not contained and explored in supervision, can generate defence mechanisms which impact directly on interactions with service users. Social workers might become directive, prescribing solutions without having fully understood a situation, or demonstrate rigidity in not exploring possible alternatives. They might withdraw, characterised by a limited use of self and avoidance of a service user's feelings and difficulties. They might avoid challenge in the hope of being liked.

Social workers will bring particular practice orientations to their work (Braye and Preston-Shoot, 2016). Thus:

- A technical orientation emphasises action underpinned by accurate legal knowledge, for which access to the latest guidance and influential case law is essential. The decision to make is whether situations of need or protection meet the legal criteria for intervention. The emphasis is on doing things right.
- A needs orientation seeks to understand people's experience. Intervention enacts obligations society owes to vulnerable people, for which needs are matched with resources or services.
- A rights orientation prioritises how the law confers or limits rights for people who use services. Action seeks to promote people's rights in relation to agency practice and in other areas of their lives. Rights are the guiding principle of decision making.
- A moral orientation sees practice as driven by ethical frameworks and goals, where the emphasis is on doing right things.
- A procedural orientation focuses on employers' policies and procedures for implementing the legal rules. Action is based on guidance from managers. Social workers work within but may not challenge organisational decision making.

These orientations may offer relevant contributions to understanding a case but, by virtue of being dominant knowledge-in-use and attitudes-in-use, other ways of viewing the situation may receive insufficient attention, with the result that needs and risks are given insufficient weight. Once again, supervision is crucial, alongside personal reflection, for enabling social workers to question and critically appraise how values, beliefs and experiences influence perspectives on legal options, assessment, need and risk.

Learning from case outcomes

Social workers might fully meet the standards of good practice outlined earlier but nonetheless fail to achieve a good case outcome. Equally, however, there are occasions when practice, and the management of practice, falls short of these standards. Public policy has therefore focused on learning lessons.

In England, Wales and Northern Ireland **Domestic Homicide Reviews** may be commissioned by a Community Safety Partnership to learn lessons regarding how agencies worked together to safeguard victims of domestic abuse, where someone aged 16 or over has died as a result of violence, abuse or neglect by a member of the same household or someone to whom they were related and/or at some point in an intimate relationship (section 9, Domestic Violence, Crime and Victims Act 2004). The focus is on learning lessons and the review is not, therefore a disciplinary inquiry. Once commissioned, a review panel is formed and terms of reference set. Agencies produce individual management reviews, critical analyses of individual and organisational practice, and its context. An overview report writer pulls together the learning from these individual reviews, focusing on lessons to be learned by, and recommendations for, those agencies collectively responsible for tackling domestic violence (Home Office, 2013). The process should normally be concluded within six months, with the overview report and executive summary made publicly available.

In England, Safeguarding Adults Boards, comprising all the agencies within a local authority area with some responsibilities for adults who require care and support, must commission **Safeguarding Adults Reviews (SARs)** when an adult dies from, or has experienced serious abuse or neglect, and concern exists about how agencies worked together. SARs may also be commissioned in other circumstances involving adults with care and support needs, including the analysis of good practice, in order to appreciate the value of learning from successful work as well as from apparent failure (DH, 2014). Board members must cooperate with such reviews and comply with any reasonable request for information (Care Act 2014). Statutory guidance (DH, 2016) indicates that the methodology used should be determined by case circumstances but that SARs should analyse what individuals and agencies might have done differently to prevent harm or death so that lessons learned can be applied to future cases. The resulting reviews do not have to be published in full but Safeguarding Adults Boards must publish the findings and recommendations in their annual reports. In Wales, Adult Practice Reviews will be commissioned in similar circumstances. In Scotland, the Adult Support and Protection (Scotland) Act 2007 enables Adult Protection Committees to commission and publish Significant Case Reviews. In the absence of a comprehensive single-nation or four-country database of such reviews, researchers have published analyses of reviews, for example involving adults who self-neglect (Braye et al, 2015a, 2015b), housing providers (Parry, 2014), and adults with learning disabilities (Manthorpe and Martineau, 2015).

All four UK countries have arrangements to review outcomes involving **children and young people** although the terminology varies. In England and Wales, Local Safeguarding Children Boards must commission Serious Case Reviews (England) or Child Practice Reviews (Wales) where a child has died or been seriously harmed, abuse and/or neglect may be involved, and where there are concerns about how effectively agencies worked together (HM Government, 2015). In Northern Ireland, the Safeguarding Board commissions Case Management Reviews on the same basis (DHSSPS, 2011). In Scotland, Child Protection Committees commission Significant Case Reviews. As with SARs and Domestic Homicide Reviews, the focus is on learning lessons rather than on finding fault and apportioning blame. Consequently, reviews may be commissioned where effective working has taken place and there are positive lessons for practice to be appreciated.

Dissemination through publication of reviews where children have died or been seriously harmed varies across the four UK nations, with government policy in England being clearest that reviews will normally be published in full (HM Government, 2015). There is a balance to be struck between protecting the anonymity of families and ensuring that professionals and their organisations are held accountable, and that learning can be disseminated and used to inform future practice. Reviews of reviews have been published in Northern Ireland (Devaney et al, 2013), Scotland (Vincent and Petch, 2012) and England (for example, Brandon et al, 2012).

Reviews of reviews across children's and adult services demonstrate that findings about **practice shortcomings are**

repetitive. In summary, common themes include (Preston-Shoot, 2014):

- lack of compliance with statutory requirements and/or failure to consider options for using legal powers;
- uncertainty about the interface between different legal mandates, such as human rights and information sharing;
- poor-quality assessments, reviews and care plans;
- limited inter-agency and multi-professional cooperation, for instance around information sharing, divergent thresholds for intervention, or understanding of safeguarding roles and responsibilities;
- poor management oversight of complex cases and supervision which does not critically explore how practitioners are approaching cases;
- poor recording;
- failure to speak to and involve children and/or adults at risk, and the absence of assertive outreach and concerned curiosity or challenge;
- failure to modify assessments and interventions as new information emerges;
- failure to implement agreed action plans and to reassess in response to increasing levels of concern;
- ignorance of chronology, meaning that agencies do not have a comprehensive view of a case.

If findings and recommendations from reviews are repetitive, then arguably lessons are not being learned. The obvious question then is "Why?" One possible answer is that reviews are not being actively disseminated and used as part of a learning and service development strategy at local level. In this context, it is noteworthy that research in Scotland found active use of serious case reviews in training organised under the auspices of Adult Protection Committees (Cornish and Preston-Shoot, 2013) and that guidance for Local Safeguarding Children Boards in England and Wales (HM Government, 2015) requires that they implement a learning and service development strategy and encourage the use of case audits alongside serious case reviews to understand what case outcomes occur and why.

A second possible answer is that insufficient priority locally is being given to the use of action learning sets, research seminars, advice sessions and case study groups where different types of knowledge, including reviews, can promote reflection and facilitate problem solving. Such thinking time can enable practitioners and managers to consider the effectiveness of interventions, the emotions aroused by a case, and the impact of policy, legal, organisational and professional contexts.

A third possible answer is that reviews have mainly adopted a forensic, technical description of what occurred, often uncovering departures from best practice but without answering the question of why practice unfolded as it did. For example, reviews often fail to identify practitioners' feelings and emotions about working with particular individuals and situations, and therefore the impact on relational interactions. The focus has been on what individuals and agencies might or should have done differently to prevent harm or death so that lessons learned can be applied to future cases. Reviews have perhaps neglected the context in which the events described occurred, for example the organisational culture and the impact on staff and services of financial austerity, the social and political expectations and critique of social work, and the complexity of the legal rules. This critique has been applied to reviews commissioned and published in England by Local Safeguarding Children Boards (Munro, 2011; Brandon et al, 2012) and Local Safeguarding Adults Boards (Flynn et al, 2011; Ash, 2013). Practitioners and managers act in a context wider than themselves and their agencies. This context has to be understood as well.

Historically, reviews of cases where children or adults have died or been seriously harmed as a result of abuse and neglect have adopted the same process of individual management reviews and overview reports, as used in Domestic Homicide Reviews. More recently, responding to the critique of the reviews, different methodologies have been used, including a systems approach (Fish et al, 2009) and a significant incident learning process (Clawson and Kitson, 2013). These approaches seek to understand systemically the working environment and its context, for example by focusing on key episodes within cases and bringing together those practitioners and managers involved in learning events where time is devoted to reflecting critically on what might have influenced how scenarios unfolded.

Individual and organisational barriers to learning

How does social work learn from those incidents when the unthinkable happens? Dissecting examples of institutional abuse and neglect of service users (for examples, see Preston-Shoot, 2014) uncovers a loss of people's humanity; their needs and wellbeing are devalued and they cease to be a focus of moral concern. Organisations are inward-looking, where power is used to stifle criticism and challenge; ethical considerations are sidelined. Resource pressures, combined with the complexity of the work and preoccupation with targets, are contained, even denied within the organisation, rather than escalated upwards and outwards. Meaningful mechanisms of holding managers and senior executives accountable are absent.

Facilitators of learning

Ethical practice is not the responsibility only of front-line practitioners and managers. Ethics are everyone's responsibility within an organisation. Knowledge, including that derived from research, should be valued and senior managers should engage with practitioners' lived experience of work and service users' lived experience of service delivery. Complaints procedures and whistle-blowing procedures should be seen as valuable additional sources of learning, alongside case reviews that incorporate understanding of the working environment and context. Supervision should be challenging as well as supportive, focusing on the quality of the work and the emotions and issues that are generated. Finally, legal rules need to provide service users and their families with adequate redress when failures of a duty of care arise.

Chapter summary

1 Mistakes are inevitable and security has costs and not only benefits. So, in the frame of appropriate error-prevention systems, social workers should pay special attention to latent errors and risks, find immediate measures to repair and limit harm and learn to prevent similar events in the future.

2 Exploration and experimentation are needed when previous attempts made using ordinary and normal strategies have failed.

3 Being wrong is an unpleasant emotional experience but it may lead to a constant and productive tension to maximise learning and minimise harm.

4 When ethical dilemmas and conflicts of interests arise, the supreme interest of the wellbeing of service users comes first. Throughout the world, codes of ethics help and guide social workers in these circumstances in order to reduce harm and risks for service users. Some of these documents also highlight the importance of reflection and constructive criticism among colleagues.

5 Legal, ethical and professional responsibilities are specifically codified across England, Wales, Scotland and Northern Ireland in case of mistakes or negative outcomes.

FOUR

Questions and narratives: basic tools for enhancing learning from professional mistakes

Learning outcomes

After this chapter you will be able to:

1 ask 'smart questions';
2 find a 'critical friend' who can offer external perspectives to extend personal reflective capacity;
3 have an overview on reflective frameworks, start using some of them and 'handcraft' new, more effective and tailor-made tools;
4 choose the most appropriate of the many different strategies for reflective writing according to goal and context;
5 use concise reflective writing as an essential, effective and practicable strategy even when working conditions make it hard to find time for structured reflection;
6 appreciate and start using different forms of metaphors, visual or written, in order to gain a holistic and deeper understanding of significant events so as to better nurture reflective practice.

Introduction

The last two chapters of this book are focused on **tools and strategies** that are available in order to improve the quality of reflection and reflective practice. This chapter presents some techniques and strategies helpful at an individual level (or in a dyadic situation) and the final chapter presents tools to be used in cooperation with other people or the entire organisation where the social workers are employed.

The quantity of tools and strategies available in literature is really huge. The ones presented here have been selected with a special focus on mistakes and failures in social work and according to their capacity to improve professional practice.

The role of **questions** is vital in any process of reflection. When people reflect they are doing nothing but asking questions of themselves. Choosing the appropriate questions is of great importance to orientate the eyes of the mind in the most fruitful direction and consequently bring the person's attention to some selected and crucial aspects of the event under scrutiny.

As the Nobel Prize winner for literature Naguib Mahfouz is reported to have said, 'you can tell whether a man is clever by his answers. You can tell whether a man is wise by his questions' (Gelb, 1996, p 96). So, since the 'right' questions are so important for learning from experience as well, and it is not easy to formulate them, there are a lot of **frameworks** developed with the purpose of making reflective practitioners 'wiser', that is to say, to enhance and deepen their reflection. They are formed by lists of questions whose purpose is to lead people to reflect on and explore the experience in detail and in areas where usually they are not looking for the solutions to their problems.

In this chapter, Gibbs' (1988) reflective cycle is described, as well as its main stages: (1) description, (2) feelings, (3) evaluation, (4) analysis, (5) conclusion, (6) action plan – and the many questions (more than 30) aimed to submit an event to a sort of 'x-ray' in order to grasp its full meaning and implications for future action. Other reflective frameworks constructed for the same purpose are also presented. With or without the use of questions, telling stories of professional errors is an indispensable tool for reflecting on these kinds of events and to understand their meaning. The role of narrative is significant both as a form of interior dialogue and as a story told by someone face to face. Each of these modes allows us to explore the past, to explain the present and direct action towards the future. Any area of personal or professional life may be subject to such a mode of investigation.

Reflective writing, which is when someone writes with the purpose of reflecting, is described and its opportunities, limits and forms (divided into two main categories: analytical and creative) are highlighted. Analytical strategies include, for example, journal writing, dialogical writing, critical incident analyses (dialogue with questions and answers using the reflective frameworks mentioned earlier), 'making a case' (with the goal of exploring alternative ways of looking at the event examined), SWOT analysis (focused on strengths, weaknesses, opportunities and threats) and others. Creative strategies also involve the emotional side of experiences and embrace writing a letter that will not be sent, writing to another person or as the other, writing as a journalist, writing a story, a fairy tale or a poem inspired by the event, drawing mind maps and others. Some strategies and suggestions for reflective writing when there is not so much time (a very common condition among social workers) are also offered in this chapter, where a specific section is dedicated to the **reflective journal** in consideration of its importance.

Finally, more **creative and 'artistic' techniques** (like audio and video recording, pictures and others) are briefly described. In fact, many forms of creativity and even arts may enhance the quality of reflection and reflective practice.

The art of asking questions

The essence of any process of reflection is made of internal dialogues that are constantly animated and nourished by questions. They are often even more important than answers because the former are useful in a wider variety of circumstances but the latter are much more situational. Even if it sounds like a paradox, it is true that there are a lot of good answers around, but good questions appear rarely and consequently are more precious.

It seems that Oscar Wilde said: 'Everyone can give an answer; it takes a genius to raise real questions' (Ravasi, 1996). The famous writer stressed the cognitive value inherent in 'smart' questions since they allow the selection of those particular aspects that make it possible to build the ultimate sense of what happened and guide this process within the informational complexity and density of the experience.

What is a 'smart' question? Who asks and answers it? What is it about? And how are good questions formulated? This first section tries to reply to these inquiries.

First, a smart question is something that puzzles, one to which it is not known immediately what to say but that leads to searching and thinking, maybe after exclaiming: "This is really a good question!" But a good question really goes to the bottom of the issue and does not abandon the thinker in a desert because in its formulation there are some hidden suggestions helping and guiding the search. According to Solomon Ibn Gabirol as cited by Johnson (2003, p 158) 'a wise man's question contains half the answer'. A similar message is included in the quotation by Fincher and Petre (2004, p 21) from Isaac and Michael (1982, p 219), when they say that 'a question well stated is a question half answered'.

A good question may be described using two images. It is like a ship sailing seas and exploring distant lands where its sailors have never been before and may find treasures and magic items, that is, as in some myths and fairy tales, something that may be able to successfully resolve difficult situations. But smart questions also metaphorically bring light into the darkness and help to explore unknown areas that previously were in shadow and where solutions for problems may be found. Reflection is often carried out where investigation has been already undertaken extensively without any important outcome, so smart questions are able to bring to light new spaces where maybe the key is to be found, as in the following funny story by Watzlawick (1983, p 31):

> Under a street lamp there stands a man, slightly intoxicated, who is searching for something. In the lighted area he searches over and over. A policeman comes along, asks him what he is looking for, and the man answers, "My keys." Now they both search. After a while the policeman wants to know whether the man is sure that he lost his keys there, and the

latter answers, "No, not here, back there – but there it is much too dark.

Good questions are able to generate knowledge because they are vital in connecting, recalling and searching for old, lost (in fact some details are almost forgotten and not considered in previous reflection) and new information. The resulting deeper understanding is similar to that achieved by social workers and their service users during interviews, no matter if these are for information gathering, decision making or therapeutic focused (Kadushin and Kadushin, 2013). The ability to make appropriate and well-stated questions may lead to a positive outcome, such as a successful helping process. But on the way to this result it is important to build a common understanding of the situation between the parts involved and good questions have a central role in attaining this result.

Second, reflection and reflective practice may be considered at three levels: **personal**, **dyadic** (one-to-one) and with a multiplicity of people in **groups** or even in **organisations**. The last of these dimensions will be examined in the next chapter, while the first and the second are considered here.

According to Thompson and Thompson (2008) everybody needs to have some time to think quietly on their own for five main reasons: to manage work pressure, to promote self-awareness, to be a free thinker (and able to depart from routine and any ready-made recipe on what is right or wrong, or how to implement it), to have so-called 'helicopter vision' (that is, a broader picture of where to place the goals, activities and results of everyday practice), and, finally, to gain clarity and focus. Being alone for reflection is highly productive but sometimes reflection in pairs may maximise the potential of learning from experience. A facilitator may give great support in this process and can be called supervisor, mentor, practice teacher, tutor, coach or peer (in this case, a colleague or a friend) who formally or informally, mutually or in the context of a complementary exchange, supports the learning process from experience.

Taylor (2010, pp 59–60) describes the role of what he calls a **'critical friend'** who:

can offer external perspectives to extend your reflective capacity. 'Critical' in this sense does not mean criticising, but being prepared to ask important questions and make tentative suggestions to unseat previous perceptions, to find other possibilities and insights.

A critical friend is chosen by you as someone you trust and respect, to assist you with your reflection. In this way the relationship is akin to mentorship, although with time and trust a delegated clinical supervisor could also fill this role. Because it requires professional respect and confidentiality, a critical friendship is initiated ideally by the person requiring guidance, and not as a delegated responsibility to a relative stranger working in the organisation.

The role of a critical friend is to listen and respond to your reflections about clinical incidents and to assist you in making some sense of them. A critical friend realises that they are not meant to be the person with answers to every dilemma that you might raise; rather, the role is to encourage you to find the answers yourself. By a well-timed question or a spontaneous supportive comment, a critical friend provides the necessary support and stimulation for you to be the main 'sense-maker' of your reflections.

It is clear that in this dyadic interrelation there is no space for useless blame and those who are recounting their stories, thoughts and emotions have to feel they are safe and not at risk of suffering any shame resulting from sharing their experiences. Without any doubt, mistakes and failures are the most difficult things to talk about and while doing this, consciously or unconsciously, it is easier to delete some shameful but also useful details. Acceptance of whatever comes out and active listening are crucial. The freer the tellers feel the deeper they can go into this learning process.

In this context the 'critical friend' stimulates telling stories from practice and, while listening, asks for more details on the 'who, when, what, where, why and how' of a particular critical situation, as well as of the feelings and emotions aroused. Further and more focused questions are very useful. 'Critical friends' can formulate questions of their own or use some of the reflective frameworks described in the next section. In both cases, their feedback is of great importance in helping social workers to reframe descriptions of events and find new connections and understandings.

On what is it most fruitful to pose questions? Literature on **critical incident** analysis provides interesting answers to this enquiry. First developed in aviation and health care, and focused on 'ineffective behaviour' (Flanagan, 1954; Green Lister, 2012), that is on mistakes and failures, the concept of 'critical incident' was probably first defined in the frame of so-called 'critical incident technique' developed by Flanagan (1954, p 327), who gave the following description:

> The critical incident technique consists of a set of procedures for collecting direct observations of human behaviour in such a way as to facilitate their potential usefulness in solving practical problems and developing broad psychological principles. The critical incident technique outlines procedures for collecting observed incidents having special significance and meeting systematically defined criteria.
>
> By an incident is meant any observable human activity that is sufficiently complete in itself to permit inferences and predictions to be made about the person performing the act. To be critical, an incident must occur in a situation where the purpose or intent of the act seems fairly clear to the observer and where its consequences are sufficiently definite to leave little doubt concerning its effects.

Later definitions in social work, and especially in social work education, are focused on a specific set of actions and their importance for the person who performed them: 'critical incidents are reflections based on analysis of the practice where the individual has taken some action and whatever he or she does has important consequences either for him or herself, the service users, others involved or all of the players' (Thomas, 2004, p 104) or, in short, 'any occurrence which was significant to a person for whatever reason' (Green Lister, 2012, p 108) and from which the professional wants to learn (Fook and Gardner, 2007). Concretely, this means to stop and reflect on an episode in which a mistake or a wrong decision was made or a risk was taken and it paid or didn't pay off. But 'critical incidents' may also be personal events, when something was done well or went better than expected, or other situations, such as when pressure, lack of confidence or support, as well as worry for service users have been felt (Green Lister, 2012; Knott and Spafford, 2013). For the many reasons described in the previous chapter, mistakes and failures are the most promising area to look into for critical incidents to reflect on. Since they are always the result of a chain of events, sometimes it is not easy to isolate a single episode from a complex stream of several happenings. Nevertheless, the need to find a form of simplification leads to segmenting the continuum in an operation similar to when the long story of a TV serial is cut into many episodes to be broadcast separately and in sequence. Driving forces and restraining factors (that is, any element which makes a mistake respectively more or less likely to occur) can be identified in any single 'episode' of the professional story and, once identified, they may lead to important learning on how to prevent mistakes in the future.

How to find good questions for an effective reflective practice? Practitioners may formulate 'smart questions' or use predefined questions. This second option will be described in the next section of this chapter referred to as reflective frameworks. The first choice is a sort of art even if everybody can learn it. As suggested by Knott and Spafford (2013, p 29), the start of this process comes from the use of the so-called 5WH formula (who, what, when, where, why and how) as well as from the detailed examination of any personal previous encounters with good questions: 'what is the best question that you have been asked [...]? Why was it a good question? Have you asked the same question of other people? What was the response?'

Going back to the image of the ship, one of two metaphors at the beginning of this section, every voyage needs clarity of destination ('When a man does not know what harbour he is making for, no wind is the right wind'; Seneca, 1979, p 163) and, similarly, it is important to have clarity on what is the most important thing that is being looked for during the process of reflection: for example, increased awareness on values, the recovery of information that had not been given particular weight in the understanding of something that went wrong, or the search for new options for action?

Questions arise especially when people meet something unexpected and they try to find new information and use what is already known to create links that may give a meaning to the unfamiliar situation. So, during any formulation of smart questions, it is important to look for connections between what is already known and what is just glimpsed at a distance, between what has already been done and what can still be done. Snyder (2003) developed an interesting model to help students (in classroom or while studying books) to ask smart questions for a better understanding of the issue of study. This model is thought to increase knowledge in training and education but it appears useful also for investigating reflexively critical incidents and can be adapted for creating questions on any happening. **Knowledge-generating questions** may be grouped in three levels: (1) general understanding, (2) insertion of the event into the existing framework of previous experiences and knowledge, (3) new directions of action. The full list of the questions for developing a rich and deep interior reflective dialogue is as follows. Level 2 and point 3.1 are left in their original form by Snyder (2003, pp 2–3), the others have some slight changes:

level 1 – general understanding

1. definitions and clarifications: how do you define/label this specific critical incident? what does this incident mean? what more general phenomenon is this incident a specific and concrete example of?
2. contextual: how was this incident shaped by the specific moment when it happened? where did this originate and why? who were the main subjects involved?

3. analysers: what parts of the incidents make up the whole and what does each part do? how do the parts contribute to the whole? how is this organised and why is it organised this way? what are the most important features of this?

level 2 – existing framework of previous experiences and knowledge

1. comparatives: how is this the same as that? how is this different from that? how are these more or less similar? what is the opposite of this?
2. casuals: what factors caused this to happen? which of these factors is sufficient? which contributing? which probable? on what grounds can we eliminate possible causes or explanations?
3. evaluation: why do you like or dislike this? how strong is the case that this is correct/wrong? what criteria are best for judging this? what is the best order or priority for these things and why? what is the strongest argument against this?

level 3 – new directions of action

1. counterfactuals: how would this change if X happened? how would things be different if X had not happened? how would things be different if X happened to a greater (or lesser) degree?
2. extenders (synthesisers): how can we apply the learning from this to this set of circumstances? what can we predict because of this? what actions can be added to this? what might happen if you added this to that?

This list of questions is different from the reflective frameworks of the next section because it needs to be much more adapted and defined according to the specific critical incident rather than to be used rigidly as most of the reflective frameworks need to be.

A similar purpose can be found in the work of Jones (2013), who described the **stages** in Table 4.1 to be used by social work students to build critical questions during their study.

Table 4.1: Stages towards asking critical questions (Jones, 2013, p 8)

Question type	Description	Attributes
fundamental	What do I think/ know about X?	describing, underpinning points with quotations
connecting	How does X relate to Y and Z?	judging, balancing different perspectives, identifying a major contender in the debate
hypothesis	If X relates to Y and Z then A	consolidation, creativity, positioning a new perspective
critical	How can I defend my argument in evaluating X, Y, Z and A?	contemplation, lateral thinking, conceptualisation of micro and macro debates and posing insightful explanations, solutions and/or challenges

Experienced social workers, and students, can find benefits for their reflective explorations in their experiences when they ask themselves questions built according to the types proposed by Jones. In addition, and since this book is focused on mistakes, it seems convenient to mention the concept of **deficit-based and strength-based questions** as described by Ghaye (2008, p 4):

> Also we have positive questions. When we focus on problems, this can so easily be the problem. By this, I mean that when we start to enquire into our problems, we begin to construct a world in which problems are central. They become the dominant realities that burden us every day. To ask questions about our failings is to create a world in which failing is the focal point. Deficit-based questions lead to deficit-based conversations, which in turn lead to deficit-based patterns of action. Yet we can flip this over and apply the same logic more positively. By asking ourselves positive questions, we may bring forth future action of far greater promise. Positive questions invite positive action.

In the previous chapters the potentiality of reflecting on mistakes was extensively described but, nevertheless, the negative impact of looking at failures and ignoring their potentiality to lead to successful intervention for the service users is evident. Somehow the two approaches can be combined transforming questions as Ghaye proposed in Table 4.2.

Table 4.2: Deficit-based and strength-based questions (Ghaye, 2008, p 203)

Deficit-based questions	Strength-based questions
1 Think of a problem that you tackled at work this week.	1 Think of a success that you achieved at work this week.
2 What were the causes of the problem?	2 What contributed to the success?
3 What needs to stop in order to 'fix' the problem?	3 What do you need to keep doing to create further success?
4 What is the one behaviour you will need to change, and how far can you do it?	4 What is the one behaviour you need to keep, and how will you keep doing it?

The comparative table on deficit-based and strength-based questions shows clearly how questions may orientate the perspective and even the answers, they involve mind and heart in a search that cannot be mechanical but needs the appropriate time and space. Questions are not for people who are in a hurry and want to find recipes for perfect and successful interventions. As the poet Rilke (1945, p 21) suggests in the following lines, they involve more than reasoning and require more than a scientific and distant approach.

> I should like to beg you earnestly to have patience with all unsolved problems in your heart and to try to love the questions themselves like locked rooms, or books that are written in a foreign tongue. Do not search now for the answers, which cannot be given you, because you could not live them. That is the point, to live everything. Now you must live

your problems. And perhaps gradually, without noticing it, you will live your way into the answer some distant day.

Reflective frameworks

Even if it could seem too simplistic, it is correct to say that reflective frameworks are sets of questions developed to help and guide reflection. There are many of them in the literature and others have been built in some professional contexts without being standardised and disseminated.

The frameworks included in this section have been selected and ordered using the dimensions **simple/complex** and **generic/specific**. In the first case the number of questions is directly proportional to the complexity of the tool, in the second the instrument can be applied to any kind of situation or, on the contrary, to some specific fields, like, for example, social work with families or learning from mistakes. In any case, there is nothing intangible in reflective frameworks and they can be changed and adapted in order to adjust them to specific personal, professional or organisational needs to be a better guide to reflective processes. What was written in the previous section on the importance of building 'smart' questions is confirmed here and the invitation to 'handcraft' new, more effective and tailor-made tools is also reaffirmed. The hammer suitable for a small hand will not be good for a hand that is bigger or with a particular shape. It is the same for a tool – it is more effective if it is in tune with personal and environmental features. So the frameworks displayed in these pages can be used as they are or can be a good start for developing other more personalised frameworks. Readers can find here a reasonable variety of material to use for this purpose.

The first of these tools is that developed by Terry **Borton** (1970, pp 93–101) for students. Its simplicity is likely to be the reason of its success. The three questions **'what'**, **'so what'**, **'now what'** are respectively thought to be organised and appropriate ways of 'increasing awareness', 'evaluating intention' and 'experimenting with new behaviour'. They are the basis for more specific questions like, for example (Rolfe et al, 2001):

- what is the problem? what did I do? what were the consequences for the user?
- so what does the event teach me? so what could I have done to make it better?
- now what do I have to do to make things better? now what do I have to do to feel better?

Borton's 'what, so what, now what' is included in the **question-based techniques for reflection–on–action** described by Thompson and Thompson (2008). They also suggest using the following focuses for other opportunities of reflection:

- Good/Bad. What went well today/this week? What didn't?
- Erase/Rewind. If I could have the time back, would I have done things differently?
- Why did I do that? Can I identify what informed my practice in this instance?
- Spot check. Do I feel in control of my workload? Could I explain my aims and objectives in my fields of responsibility if called on to do so now?
- Humble pie. Have I been challenged today/this week and learned a lesson from it?
- Making a difference. What part did I play in promoting change today/this week and learned a lesson from it? Was it positive or negative change? At what level? (Thompson and Thompson, 2008, p 100)

The same authors proposed **question-based techniques** for reflection not only after an intervention or an event but also before (**reflection-for-action**) and during (**reflection-in-action**). The three simple tools suggested for decision making (that is, for-action) nurtured by a well-focused reflection on previous similar experiences are based on some easy questions like:

1. what are you trying to achieve? how are you going to achieve it? how will you know when you have achieved it?
2. what are you trying to achieve? what is it that will contribute to the achievement of that aim? what action needs to be taken to bring about what has been highlighted when the second question has been answered? A tree diagram with three levels has to be used to give a visual representation of the plan built by answering the three key-questions.
3. the word 'why' is used to formulate questions as shown in the following example (related to a situation of risk of aggression) where it is embedded in an internal dialogue or in a conversation with someone who, for example, has the role of the 'reflective friend' described in the previous section (Thompson and Thompson, 2008, p 84):
4. 'Why am I feeling anxious about working with Mr Walters?
5. I am worried about the potential for violence.
6. Why am I worried about the potential for violence?
7. Last time I went there he was aggressive towards me.
8. Why was he aggressive towards me?
9. He seemed to think I was intending to report him to the police because I was aware he was using illegal drugs.
10. Why would he assume that?
11. He seems to see me as an authority figure. Perhaps he doesn't understand my role.
12. Why wouldn't he understand my role?
13. Perhaps I didn't explain it clearly enough to him. If I want him to avoid being aggressive towards me again, I will need to make sure he has a good understanding of my role.'

Reflection-in-action is probably the most complex of the three kinds of reflections highlighted by Thompson and Thompson because it integrates activity and thought simultaneously. In fact, ongoing actions have to flow and cannot be interrupted by too much complex thinking. In the same way, for example, pianists cannot think: 'now I have to press this piano key, then the other, then quicker ...' in the middle of a concert. If they do so their performance is irretrievably ruined. Nevertheless, the circular flow of actions and feedback is positively enhanced by simple and well-focused questions referred to as the so-called 3H (head, heart, habit) or, similarly, by the triad 'think–feel–do' recalling the wholeness and interactions of mind, feelings and actions. It is important not to forget that social work is a risky profession for workers and users, so in difficult situations it is important to give a prompt **risk** assessment and reaction answering questions on: 'whether to act, when to act, whether we have enough information on which to base an informed decision' (Thompson and Thompson, 2008, p 90).

After these examples of tools based on a few and well-focused questions (even if they are inevitably limited in the breadth of vision offered) and before presenting two examples of reflective frameworks for specific fields, the following part of this section will present the '7+5' questions of Ingram et al (2014) on critical reflection and reflexivity, the 10 and 17 questions for critical incident analysis of, respectively, Thomas (2004) and Green Lister and Crisp (2007), and the most complex, Gibbs' reflective cycle (1988) and the technical, practical and emancipatory reflection frameworks of Beverley Joan Taylor (2010). These tools are useful to understand in depth any experience in professional life but may be of special interest to social workers who want to fully and specifically understand their mistakes. The many questions of this chapter are well suited to discover the reasons for what 'went wrong'. There are different focuses in the frameworks of these pages so everybody can choose the one that is most suitable to their sensibilities and research purposes.

To begin with, when they talk about reflective social work practice, Ingram et al (2014) use (critical) reflection and reflexivity and distinguish the first from the second. The term reflectivity may be substituted by **critical reflection** when the search is focused on a deeper understanding of what is behind events, actions and thoughts in terms of influence from cultural and historical contexts, as well as personal life experiences. This distinction between the two worlds may lead to the different lists of reflective questions in Table 4.3.

Table 4.3: Questions to prompt reflection and reflexivity (adapted from Ingram et al, 2014, p 30)

	Questions for critical reflection	Questions for reflexivity
Event	What happened?	How did I influence what happened?
Purposes or causes	Why did it happen?	Why did I behave in that way?
Feelings	How was I feeling?	Why might I have felt the way I did during the situation, and now, when reflecting on it?
Assumptions and influence of identity	What were my assumptions? What informed these assumptions?	How has who I am affected my view of what happened, my values, opportunities and life choices, and subsequently my reflection?
Changes	What needs to change? What can I do next time?	What beliefs or ways of challenging my assumptions will allow me to look at this from others' perspectives?

Developed as a tool for practice teachers in social work, the following two frameworks may enhance a deep **analysis of critical incidents**.

The first was elaborated by Thomas (2012, p 107) and has the following instructions and questions:

- Give a brief outline of the situation, what happened, who was involved, where it took place. Include any relevant issues of oppression or discrimination that you were aware of.
- Describe what you did or said, what action you took and what the response was from others?
- How were you feeling at the time and how do you think others were feeling?
- What were the main challenges for you?
- What went well and what did you do to enable this?
- What underpinning knowledge and theories did you use? What methods of intervention did you use? How where these informed by research and evidence-based practice?
- What values underpinned the work and how did you demonstrate or convey these?
- What value conflicts were you aware of and how did you deal with these?
- If you were undertaking a similar piece of work again is there anything you would do differently? If so, what? If not, why not?
- What do you think you learned from the work?
- What have you learned from reviewing the situation and your practice within it? (The question is posed after the incident has been discussed in small groups).

Green Lister and Crisp (2007, pp 49–50) formulated the following **17 questions** and tested them with social work students engaged in their field practice. Devised for **anti-oppressive practice**, this framework helps in reflectively reviewing critical incidents, responses to them (in terms of related dilemmas as well), outcomes and learning.

1. Account of the incident
   What happened, where and when; who was involved?
   What was your role/involvement in the incident?

What was the context of this incident, e.g. previous involvement of yourself or other from this agency with this client/client group?
What was the purpose and focus of your contact/intervention at this point?

2. Initial responses to the incident
What were your thoughts and feelings at the time of this incident?
What were the responses of other key individuals to this incident? If not known, what do you think these might have been?

3. Issues and dilemmas highlighted by this incident
What practice dilemmas were identified as a result of this incident?
What are the values and ethical issues which are highlighted by this incident?
Are there implications for inter-disciplinary and/or inter-agency collaborations which you have identified as a result of this incident?

4. Learning
What have you learned, e.g. about yourself, relationships with others, the social work task, organisational policies and procedures?
What theory (or theories) has (or might have) helped develop your understanding about some aspect of this incident?
What research has (or might have) helped develop your understanding about some aspect of this incident?
How might an understanding of the legislative, organisational and policy contexts explain some aspects associated with this incident?
What future learning needs have you identified as a result of this incident? How might these be achieved?

5. Outcomes

What were the outcomes of this incident for the various participants?

Are there ways in which this incident has led (or might lead to) changes in how you think, feel or act in particular situations?

What are your thoughts and feelings now about this incident?

One of the most popular reflective frameworks in health and social professions is **Gibbs' reflective cycle** (Gibbs, 1988), developed from Kolb's idea of the ERA (Experience, Reflection, Action) cycle mentioned in chapter one of this book. Figure 4.1 shows the global structure of this tool and its six stages.

Figure 4.1: Structure of Gibbs' reflective cycle

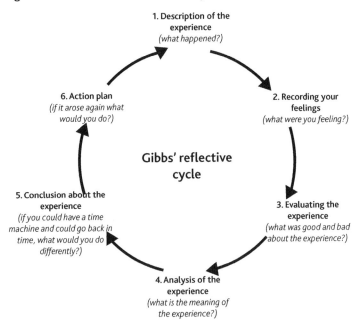

Source: Adapted from Gibbs, 1988

Metaphorically Gibbs' reflective cycle can be imagined like a wardrobe with six drawers. On the front of each drawer there is a label (description, feelings, evaluation and so on) and a key-question (what happened? what were you thinking and feeling? what was good and bad about the experience? and so on) and inside there are more detailed questions to go deeper into reflection. The first two stages are descriptive of external (events) and internal (feelings) 'facts' without making any judgement or trying any conclusion. These provide the scope for the following stages (evaluation and analysis), when the 'good' and the 'bad' of the critical incident under scrutiny are explored in order to draw out their meaning. The last two stages are vital to bring the learning into the plan of a new action. First, the workers have to imagine what different and better action they could have performed. It is like answering the question: if you could have a time machine and could go back in time, what would you do differently? Of course, time travel is impossible but thinking about it is a sort of mental experiment that can help in answering the final key-question: if this issue arose again what would you do?

Gibbs' reflective cycle is an effective tool for personal reflection or for thinking things over with a colleague (this 'reflective friend' may ask and insist if a question is not fully answered or is skipped). It may be used in speaking or in writing as well. For all these uses, Tate (2013, pp 90–2) adapted Gibbs' original work as follows:

1. Description of the experience (what happened?)
   [...]
   • Describe what happened in your own words using the first person ...
   • How did you act during the experience?
   • What were your thoughts during the experience?
   [...]

2. Recording your feelings (what were you feeling?)
   [...]
   • How did you feel, i.e. emotions (positive and negative) and other thoughts?
   • At what point in the experience did the emotion start?

• Did you notice any physical symptoms associated with the emotion?
[...]

3. Evaluating the experience
   [...]
   • Why did I interpret the situation in the way I did?
   • What other interpretations might there be?
   • Why did I act/intervene the way I did?
   • What were the consequences of my actions for myself/others involved?
   • How are negative feelings/assumptions holding me back?
   • How did positive feelings influence what happened?
   • How did negative feelings and fears influence what happened?
   • What assumptions did I make, about myself, about others?
   • What did others involved do, think, feel?

4. Analysis of the experience
   [...]
   • What might I have done differently? What might have been the outcome?
   • How might I put aside the features that are holding me back?
   • What do I need to learn more about, and how will I learn it? (This includes background reading)
   • How can I apply new learning and strategies?

5. Conclusion about the experience
   [...]
   • What have I learned from the experience (about self, others, issues)?
   • How has my understanding developed?
   • How will I apply it another time?

- What do I need to work on – and how will I work on it?

6. Action plan
   [...]
   - What is your goal?
   - What steps do you need to take to achieve your goal?
   - What resources do you need to achieve your goal?
   - What is the time frame for each of these steps?
   - What will be the outcome of each step?

It is interesting to note that originally the third stage (evaluation) was focused on the questions 'What was good/bad about that?', which looks better for reflecting on a mistake and helps to focus on both the positive and the negative implications of any kind of event, since failures and successes are never 'pure' bad or good critical incidents.

Considering the differences between **practical reflection and emancipatory reflection** (the first is related to interpretative knowledge, the second leads to action to gain freedom from oppressive forces and what is taken for granted), Beverley John Taylor (2010) suggests several questions and grouped them respectively into three (experiencing, interpreting, learning) and four (constructing, deconstructing, confronting, reconstructing) stages. The questions for starting both kinds of reflection are the same, but then the processes go in different directions according to different aims. 'As the main intentions of practical interests are to describe and explain human interaction, they are concerned with interpretation and explanation through practical reflection, which in turn creates interpretive knowledge' (2010, p 127). On the other hand, emancipatory reflection is interested in highlighting the practice constraints in any professional action and in identifying what prevents the worker from practising effectively.

Table 4.4 contains a comparative picture of all the questions proposed by Taylor and makes it possible to conduct a detailed exploration combining the benefits of the two different forms

Table 4.4: Practical and emancipatory reflection – comparative table

	Practical reflection	Emancipatory reflection	
Experiencing	• What was happening? • When was it happening? • Where was it happening? • What was the setting like, in terms of its smells, sounds and sights? • Why was it happening? • Who was involved? • How were you involved? • What were the outcomes of the situation? • How did you feel honestly about the situation?		**Constructing**
		It seems as if I act according to my belief that ...	**Deconstructing**
Interpreting	• What were my hopes for the practice outcomes in this story? • How were my hopes related to my ideals of what constitutes 'good' practice? • What are the sources in my life and work for my ideas and values for communicative aspects of my practice? • In what ways do I embody them now in the way I communicate at work? • What was my communicative role in this situation? • To what extent did I achieve my communicative role? • How did my interpretation of my role affect my relations with the people in the situation? • What are the shared communication norms and expectations in this situation? In other words, how did everyone else in the story interpret their roles and what did they seem to expect in the situation? • To what extent were social norms, or sets of expectations for behaviour, operating in this situation? • What system of spoken and unspoken rewards and penalties was in place to maintain and control socially accepted behaviours in this situation? • Were the usual communicative norms and sanctions altered in this situation?	• Where did the ideas I embody in my practice come from historically? • How did I come to appropriate them? In other words, how did I take them on? • Why do I continue now to endorse them in my work? • Whose interests do they serve? • What power relations are involved? • How do these ideas influence my relationships with the people in mycare? • What cultural, economic, historical, political, social and/or personal constraints are operating in this practice story?	**Confronting**

	Practical reflection	Emancipatory reflection	
Learning	• What does this scenario tell me about my expectations of myself? • What does this scenario tell me about my expectations of other people? • What have I learned from this situation? • What kinds of adaptations are possible in my work relationships? • How do I fit these new insights into my present ways of regarding communicative action in my work?	In the light of what I have discovered, how might I work differently?	Reconstructing

Source: Adapted from Taylor, 2010, pp 134–5, 151–3.

of reflection. Expectations and hopes, embodied ideas, power relations and other variables may lead to a deeper awareness and learning on how to act differently in order to make better interventions for the benefit of service users.

These frameworks are quite complex but nevertheless they allow a very detailed and in-depth analysis of professional experiences in any field of social work. These are the last 'generalist' tools proposed in this section. In fact, the final two frameworks here are specific and focused on two areas of social work: first, social work with families and, second, on mistakes in social work.

Canavan (2006, pp 282, 285) lists 10 practice principles to be followed for family support and identifies 4 questions. The principles are:

1. working in partnership with children, families, professionals and communities;
2. needs led and striving for the minimum intervention required;
3. clear focus on the wishes, feelings, safety and well-being of children;
4. reflects a strengths-based/resilience perspective;
5. strengthens informal support networks;
6. accessible and flexible incorporating both child protection and out-of-home care;
7. facilitates self-referral and multi-access referral paths;

8. involves service users and front-line providers in the planning, delivery and evaluation;
9. promotes social inclusion, addressing issues of ethnicity, disability and rural/urban communities;
10. outcomes-based evaluation supports quality services based on best practice.

The questions to be asked for each of the 10 principles in relation to any specific example of family support are:

1. What are the indicators of the achievement of the principle?
2. What level of performance is being achieved by the intervention/service/organisation?
3. What actions need to be taken to achieve the principle in practice?
4. What has been learned from trying to implement the principle?

It is clear that these four questions can be used to analyse any critical incident in any specific field of social work in the light of its related principles.

Finally, the following and last reflective framework is focused on errors and failures in social work. This framework has been built combining a part of the content of the previous chapter with some of the key-questions already mentioned in this section. Other questions, then, have been added. The division into six sections and many of the questions are clearly taken from the Gibbs' reflective cycle.

1 DESCRIPTION
It is important to write in the first person, as objectively as possible and as if you were watching the event, without judgement but reporting any insights and thoughts which emerged during the event as if they were part of the experience.

1. What happened, where and when? Who was involved? Where were you? Who else was with you? Why were you there? Were these normal/normative circumstances?
2. What were you doing? What were the other people doing?

3. What was the context of the event (for example, routine or normal)? What happened?
4. Which part in what happened did you undertake? Which part did the others undertake? What was your role in the event and what was the role of each of the others?
5. What was the purpose of the intervention/challenge?
6. What was the result?

2 FEELINGS
1. How did you feel, that is, what were your emotions (positive and negative) and thoughts?
2. What were your feelings and your thoughts immediately before the event started? During? After? Was it a usual day?
3. Were there feelings or emotions that were present at the outset of the event or during the event that may have contributed and how?
4. At what point of the experience did you specifically start to feel each of these emotions, or were they present at the outset?
5. What did the words, the interventions, the challenges and the actions of other participants make you think? How did they make you feel?
6. Were there physical reactions and symptoms associated with emotions?
7. How do you feel now when you think back to the error/failure?
8. What did the other people involved in the event do, think and feel? How do you know this?

3 ASSESSMENT
1. What would you describe as positive and what might be described as negative in the experience?
2. What specific parts of this event and the evidenced error/failure are most important for you?
3. What do you think specifically went wrong? For whom? According to which technical ideas or ethical principles?
4. What is specifically right? For whom? According to which technical ideas or ethical principles?

5. Why did you interpret the situation the way you interpreted it?

6. What other interpretations could there be?

4 ANALYSIS

1. Why did you behave the way you did?

2. What were the consequences of your actions for yourself and for others involved?

3. How do your negative feelings and your negative evaluations prevent you from rethinking the event?

4. How have your positive feelings influenced what happened?

5. How have your negative feelings and fears influenced what happened?

6. What assumptions did you make about yourself and others?

7. How did you influence what happened? Why did it happen? Why did you behave like that?

8. How did you feel? Why did you feel that way during the event and why do you feel the way you feel now when you reflect on the event?

9. What were your assumptions? What has shaped these assumptions? How has who you are affected your view of what happened, your values, opportunities and life choices, and subsequently your reflection?

10. In a very few words, what would you label this mistake? What more general failure is this error/failure a specific and concrete example of?

11. Had you made a similar error/failure in the past? When? How often? How is this different from the previous ones? What prevented you from putting a stop to the repetition of this kind of error/failure?

12. What chain of events led to the error/failure? What was the role of each of the following stages/levels?
    ○ top-level decision makers (social policies, direction, goal of general and inherent resource allocation);
    ○ line management (that is, implementation by the executive level of the strategies defined at the above level);

◦ preconditions (motivations, equipment and so on) of the subjects and factors directly involved in the implementation of social work services such as users, practitioners, material resources and so on;

◦ productive activities (when the analysed event occurred);

◦ defence systems (among the issues to be included there is the image of social workers and their service – for example, which side is the social worker perceived as being on?).

5 CONCLUSION

1. What factors caused the error/failure to happen? Which are the three most important factors?

2. How would this change if X happened? How would things be different if X had not happened? How would things be different if X happened to a greater (or lesser) intensity?

3. What needed to stop in order to fix the problem or for behaviour to change? What evidence do you have to consider these factors as relevant? How much can you eliminate or to what extent can you reduce the strength of these casual factors?

4. If you could go back in time, what would you do differently?

5. What could you have done differently? What would have been the result?

6 ACTION PLAN

1. What do you need to change? What can you do differently next time when you deal with a similar case?

2. What actions can be made to prevent this error/failure in the future? When can you do this? What can you do right now? How will you know you have fixed the problem and the same mistake will not happen again?

3. What is the goal of improvement that you can choose? What steps should you take to reach your goal? Which resources do you need to achieve your goal? How long does it take for each of these stages? What will be the result of each of these stages? How could you put aside the things that prevent you from improving?

4. What have you learned from this experience (about yourself, others and so on)? How has your understanding developed?
5. How will you apply this new understanding in the future on another occasion? What do you need to know more about and how do you plan to learn more? How can you apply new learning and strategies?
6. What do you need to work on and how will you work on it?

Table 4.5 summarises what a social worker wrote about a failure she reflected on using the framework described before. The value of reflective writing and the forms it takes will be at the centre of the next section. Here it is important to give an example of how the many questions proposed earlier may lead the exploration and search for meaning and learning.

It is clear that in the proposed synthesis some questions of the framework are not considered, as they were missing from the original report. Readers could try to identify which, among the many in the framework, would be the most important questions to ask in order to investigate the episode and enrich the final 'action plan'. It is a good exercise since it can help social workers to learn to review their reflections periodically in order to deepen their learning from mistakes. As already described in this book (chapter one), reflective practice is a circular process, not a linear one.

Table 4.5: Reflective framework on errors and failures – synthesis of a case study

Stage	Short description
1. Description	Four social workers from different services and I met to plan and coordinate our actions to support a child and his parents. We had to check what happened after the previous and first meeting. After a brief update it was clear that only a few workers had done what was planned. Mutual recriminations started when the coordinator's impatience detonated the underlying tension. The group even failed to agree a date for a third meeting.
2. Feelings	I felt and still feel discomfort and devalued. I observed anger and mutual accusation in the group and this left a sense of frustration and failure because we were not able to convey the general annoyance into something constructive.
3. Assessment	The negative aspect was the deadlock in the intervention. The positive was that many unspoken things from the first meeting emerged, but this did not allow us to overcome the impasse and move on. It is ethically bad that we were not able to do the best for our service users without any delay. At the same time we were not able to use teamwork properly.
4. Analysis	We had not worked together before on other cases. We all work in the same areas where services are still struggling to work together and create a stronger network for the community. Maybe top and line management are not committed enough to this. We also did not fully detail the specific goal of our action together at the beginning. The coordinator (the social worker of the organisation that convened the meeting) was not assertive enough. I was too shy during the meeting because of my inexperience and do not feel self-confident enough in my professional skills.
5. Conclusion	The organisation that convened the meeting should have better prepared the meeting explaining the aim more clearly right from the beginning. Lack of experience and coordination, together with weak connections between our organisations are the most important factors that caused the failure.
6. Action plan	In this and similar situations my four colleagues and I have to better understand what we want 'to take home' right from the beginning. We also have to promote better cooperation between our managements in order to create a framework where social workers can more easily know each other and work together.

Reflective writing

Reflection can be carried out on a mental and meditative level, or verbally, that is, talking to other people about an event. Then there is a further area represented by writing.

In all these cases social workers narrate, that is, they select, order and report events (Knott and Scragg, 2013). As Taylor says (2006, p 80), '**narratives** are regarded as a way of ordering the scattered and temporary dispersed events of our lives'. It is like ordering messy houses, putting things in the right place to make them available to be used in the future.

Especially in social work, 'stories matter because they can accommodate contradictions, connections and discontinuities in our everyday practice' (Frost, 2006, p 116). What is more contradictory than unexpected outcomes or, more precisely, failures, that is clashes between expectation and reality? Telling the story of a mistake is an important step in any process of replacing old and ineffective beliefs with new ones that potentially may create a better relationship between past, present and future. This is the reason why narrative methods are powerful tools for reflection and professional development.

Starting from these considerations, this section will be focused on the 'what, why and how' of reflective writings, with a final look at how to use this essential tool for reflective practice when there is little or almost no time to write.

First of all, **what is** reflective writing? It is the deliberate use of strategies of writing as a way of reflecting on and learning from experience. The purpose of learning makes this form of writing different from any others (Rolfe et al, 2001). Everywhere social workers have to write many reports and other forms of documents are an essential part of their daily tasks, but these are aimed at 'nurturing' the process of help, with special regard to organisational needs. Instead, reflective writing drives learning and, with the intent of building a genuine reflective practice, implies that any description of events is not enough but has to lead to critical reflection. This happens when questions and answers are developed, emotions and their meaning are considered, others' views are taken into account and personal beliefs and assumptions are referred to social, political norms and theoretical perspectives (Bruce, 2013).

Why is it so good to reflect in a written form? What specifically can reflective writing be useful for?

As often found in the literature (Rolfe et al, 2001; Jasper, 2003) reflective writing helps to:

- order events, thoughts and feelings related to the working practice;
- record experience in its most significant details;
- develop analytical skills, creativity and critical thinking;
- identify connections between information, integrate experience and give meaning to it.

Writing, then, is to help get out of the emotional and intellectual turmoil produced by some events, such as the ones labelled as professional errors. This happens when what is in mind goes on a sheet of paper or an electronic one and so finds structure and order. But, even if the episode under analysis does not arouse particular emotions, writing leads to the selection of the most significant features among the many characterising the experience, or, in other words, to identifying priorities within the large sea of descriptive details of an experience. This work is facilitated by the fact that the act of writing is slower than thinking or talking. If there is no selection and prioritisation of the information, too much data would have to be considered and impasse would be inevitable, similar to what happened to the main character of the fantasy short story 'Funes the Memorious' written by Borges and included in his collection *Ficciones* (1962). In this novel the main character, Ireneo Funes, gains perfect and infallible perception and memory, after a fall from a horse, and because of this transformation 'the present was almost intolerable, it was so rich and bright; the same was true of the most ancient and most trivial memories' and 'he could reconstruct all his dreams, all his fancies. Two or three times he had reconstructed an entire day. He told me: [...] *My memory, sir, is like a garbage disposal*' (Borges, 1962, p 112; original italics). Writing in detail using such prodigious ability to remember would be nonsense if one is looking for the essence of the experience and the consequent learning. Forgetfulness helps to find the meaning of an event. It is similar to what many artists do when they bring out a sculpture from a block of marble, because they 'free' it from any excess material covering the sculpture.

Selecting from memories and emotions is a fundamental step to give meaning to any experience and, then, to generalise so to be better equipped in facing the future. This means, just to remain in the metaphor offered by Borges, defeating another curse that Funes had. In fact he was:

> almost incapable of general, platonic ideas. It was not only difficult for him to understand that the generic term dog embraced so many unlike specimens of differing sizes and different forms; he was disturbed by the fact that a dog at three-fourteen (seen in profile) should have the same name as the dog at three-fifteen (seen from the front). His own face in the mirror, his own hands, surprised him on every occasion. (Borges, 1962, p 114)

This leads to the second point included in the list: to record experience in its most significant details. In fact, reflective writing helps to rescue and recover detailed memories of the event under consideration, including those that have almost been forgotten or considered unimportant (Rolfe et al, 2001). Writing close to the event, as well as being aware that the narrative is always developed in the light of subsequent experiences, reinforces this function of reflective writing that also promotes the development of analytical skills, enhances critical thinking, makes people more creative and helps them to identify innovative ways of problem solving. So it is possible to identify the assumptions governing the action and the most influential aspects of the context. New alternatives can be imagined and explored in a context of 'reflexive scepticism' that leads to an attitude of continuous research and discourages us from thinking that there is only one way of seeing things and only one good explanation for what happened (Jasper, 2003).

Finally, reflective writing helps practitioners to find connections between different ideas and develop integrated frameworks with meaning, coherence and internal harmony. Linking information that has been collected in a fragmentary way, and creating bridges between theory and practice may also lead to this result (Rolfe et al, 2001).

Despite its many benefits, why is reflective writing so little practised? What are the **obstacles**? There are many reasons preventing such a good habit from spreading: in the first place, previous negative experiences, for example when nothing positive has been found from some material written for reflective purposes, may have an effect. More often, then, social workers do not feel free and they fear that confidentiality is at risk if the wrong eyes read what they unreservedly wrote (Jasper, 2003).

However, the most important impediment is time. Two objections may be opposed to the affirmation 'I have no time!', which is more often a kind of translation of the sentence 'I have other priorities.' First, reflective writing can be challenging and unpleasant sometimes (looking in a mirror can show unpleasant things), but, as this book is trying to demonstrate, it can be particularly fruitful.

Second, writing takes too much time. In an interview a psychologist with 30 years' experience said 'you do not need so much time because you can do it between one service user and another. You can do it. You do not need so much time to write in order to reflect' (Sicora, 2010, p 100). This activity is an investment in professional development and maintains the many tools practitioners need to face their daily complex work. The ones who do not do so, claiming they are overwhelmed by urgency, seem like the lumberjack who, while in difficulty cutting down a tree with an old and worn saw, refused to stop and pick up a new instrument or sharpen the old one so to finish the work with less effort, saying that he had no time because he had to saw the trunk.

Besides, everyone can freely choose the amount of time to dedicate to writing. Even the simple and rapid strategy of summarising the working day at its end in the form of a newspaper headline can have surprising results: while choosing the appropriate words social workers would have to think and find the most significant aspects of that particular day. At the end of a month the list of these titles will give a synthetic vision and view 'from above' of what has happened in that period. Such an overview is very useful to better understand trends that often are not captured because social workers are too much taken up with routine.

So now, after these considerations on the opportunities and obstacles of reflective writing, **how** to do it? What are the main **strategies**? Rolfe et al (2001) and Jasper (2004, p 105) take account of the many available selections and divide them into two categories: **analytical** (characterised by objectivity and the attempt to stand back from the events considered) and creative (using imagination, metaphors and emotions, sometimes, in their rawest forms). Examples of the first group are: critical incident analysis, dialogical writing (creating a conversation through questions and answers), making a case (exploring the alternative perspectives on an issue), creating an ongoing record, SWOT analysis (identifying the strengths, weaknesses, opportunities and threats within an experience), using a structured reflective framework, identifying three-a-day (for example, 'Three things I have learned today are …'), page-a-day record of experiences, writing a word-limited summary. Examples of **creative** strategies are: writing an unsent letter or email, to a nominated other person (for example a close friend) or as the other person, or as a journalist, or writing poetry, a story or a review in a particular style (fantasy, science-fiction and so on.)

A form of writing not included in these lists is the professional portfolio. As stated by Rolfe et al (2001, p 64):

> an essential and critical difference between a portfolio *per se* and the strategies of reflective writing is that a portfolio is designed and constructed to portray a picture of its creator and, as such, is likely to be open to public scrutiny in some form. Whilst reflective writing may well be included in and form an essential part of a portfolio, it behoves the writer to make clear decisions as to what part of the portfolio is selected for others to read.

Bolton (2010) widens the scope of reflective writing strategies, proposing some exercises for professional development focused on a **global picture of professional life** rather than **specific critical incidents**. Here is a selection of the more significant of these strategies (Bolton, 2010, p 24).

Names

1. Write anything about your name: memories, impressions, likes, hates, what people have said, your nicknames over the years – anything.
2. Write a selection of names you might have preferred to your own.
3. Write a letter to yourself from one of these chosen names.
4. Read back to yourself with care, adding or altering positively.

Milestones

1. List the milestones of your life and/or career, do it quickly without thinking much.
2. Read back to self: delete or add, clarify or expand as you wish.
3. Add some divergent things (for example, when you first really squared up to your head of department).
4. Choose one. Write a short piece about it. If you wish, continue and write about others.
5. Read back to yourself with care, add or delete (without listening to your negative critic).

Insights

1. Write a quick list of 20 words or phrases about your work.
2. Allow yourself to write anything; everything is relevant, even the seeming insignificant.
3. Reread; underline ones which seem to stick out.
4. Choose one. Write it at the top of a fresh page. Write anything which occurs to you.

5. NOBODY [*sic*] else needs read this ever, so allow yourself to write anything.
6. You might write a poem, or an account remembering a particular occasion, or muse ramblingly. Whatever you write will be right.
7. Choose another word from your list, if you wish, and continue writing.
8. Add to your list if more occurs to you.
9. Reread with care, adding or altering, using only a positive approach.

As mentioned before, lack of time is one of the most common obstacles to reflective writing. Some strategies may help in overcoming this problem. They all request a limited number of words or characters so as to help in focusing on the most important things. Consequently a lot of time is saved in the act of writing, even if some time is needed to reflect and select the appropriate terms. In fact, the writing of a few words will be preceded by an in-depth reflection in search of the 'concentrated juice' from the experience, that is its meaning and teaching for the future. This concept (that is, reflection requires more time than writing) was also indirectly expressed by the philosopher Blaise Pascal, who is said to have written the following sentence in one of his *Lettres provinciales* in 1657: 'I have made this letter longer than usual, because I lack the time to make it short' (Wormeli, 2003, p xii). What Pascal wrote is maybe paradoxical and excessive but nevertheless reflection must mainly come before writing in any **strategy for concise reflective writing**.

For example, the Gibbs' reflective cycle is even more effective when it produces a written report with a limited number of words, as proposed in Table 4.6. The insight is focused and the final product is very rich in learning.

Table 4.6: Reflective writing using the Gibbs' reflective cycle with a limited number of words (Lia, 2014, p 5)

Steps	%	Approximate number of words for each stage of the reflection			
		1,000 word reflection	1,500 word reflection	2,000 word reflection	2,500 word reflection
1. Description	20	200	300	400	500
2. Feeling	10–20	150	225	300	375
3. Evaluation	20	200	300	400	500
4. Analysis	30	300	450	600	750
5. Conclusion	5–10	75	112	150	187
6. Action Plan	5–10	75	112	150	187

Another similar but even more extreme strategy consists in summarising an event in only 160 characters, that is the size of an SMS (Short Message Service) text used in written communications between mobile phones for years and, possibly, learning from it. In chapter two, some of these texts written by social workers during continuing education courses have been put forward in order to explore professional mistakes in social work. As mentioned earlier in this section, even giving a title to an episode of professional life, as if it were the title of an article, may be an act of in-depth reflection.

In Table 4.7 there are some examples of these two extremely concise forms of reflective writing. They were collected during a training course for social workers from different fields of activity and are related to experiences of mistakes with more or less grave consequences (in one case a service user committed suicide).

Table 4.7: Examples of extremely concise reflective writings (titles and SMS)

Title	SMS
Lonely in front of the tragic event with guilt feelings.	Elder found dead 20 days later because neighbours gave the alarm. Social worker didn't fulfil the mandate. Never be superficial in apparently easy cases.
Ifs and buts do not make history ... But you learn a lot!	Teenager in community unable to return home but against any fostering. I didn't insist. He returned to his addicted mother and he also became so. More decision!
Dialogue of the deaf.	Difficult interview. I do not like these relatives. It's useless. They do not understand. Maybe they did not listen. Maybe I have to. Well, next time I will.
The Scream by Munch.	I had not expected this. I underestimated the situation. I did not think he would express, in that way, that pain. Never assume anything.
Patient attacks the legal guardian: executioner or victim?	Poor assessment and welcome. Legal guardian assaulted by psychiatric patient. We must assess the situation carefully to avoid bad consequences.

These two strategies (SMS and title) need very little time and are especially effective to reflect not only on single events but also on what globally happened during medium to long periods. If a text message or a title is written every day or every week, at the end of the month or of the year, numerous concise writings will be available to offer a comprehensive picture of what happened in that period. This reflective material is produced easily and quickly (a few minutes a day or a week are enough) but is very rich, gives a global view of what has happened and is not too much influenced by the most recent episodes and the moment when the final reflection is carried out.

Reflective journal to learn how to navigate through the calms and storms of professional practice

The most effective and complete tool for reflective writing is the so-called learning or reflective journal. Its main purpose is to capture and look back on experience and it may be considered as a 'vehicle for reflection' Moon (2006, p 1). Moon also proposes a **definition** of this instrument and asserts that:

> by learning journal, we refer to an accumulation of material that is mainly based on the writer's processes of reflection. The accumulation is made over a period of time, not 'in one go'. The notion of 'learning' implies that there is an overall intention by the writer (or those who have set the task) that learning should be enhanced. (2006, p 2)

Similarly Holly (1988, p 78) states that:

> a journal is a record of happenings, thoughts and feelings about a particular aspect of life, or with a particular structure. A journal can record anything relative to the issue to which it pertains. So a reflective journal is like a diary of practice, but in addition includes deliberate thought and analysis related to practice.

A learning journal does not consist of a bare description of events, thoughts and emotions that, once written on paper or in an electronic file, is put away and forgotten. On the contrary, it is a sort of artefact made little by little, composed of many layers accumulated over time, whenever reading, rereading and writing more notes and reflections take place. This recording of events and experiences has to be done on an incremental basis, including commentaries and accounts, so as to identify new knowledge and learning (Jasper, 2004).

Why should social workers start their own reflective journal? Personal and professional development through reflection empowered by a written record of events and reflections is the main purpose of someone who starts keeping a learning journal. Table 4.8 contains a detailed list of the benefits of this reflective tool according to Moon (2006) and Tate (2013):

Table 4.8: Purposes of keeping reflective journals (Moon, 2006, pp 44–51; Tate, 2013, pp 58–9)

Moon (2006)	Tate (2013)
• To record experience • To facilitate learning from experience • To support understanding and the representation of the understanding • To develop critical thinking or the development of a questioning attitude • To encourage metacognition • To increase active involvement in and ownership of learning • To increase ability in reflection and thinking • To enhance problem-solving skills • As a means of assessment in formal education • To enhance reflective practice • For reasons of personal development and self-empowerment • For therapeutic purposes or as a means of supporting behaviour change • To enhance creativity • To improve writing • To improve or give 'voice'; as a means of self-expression • To foster communication and to foster reflective and creative interaction in a group • To support planning and progress in research or a project • As a means of communication between one learner and another	**Process reasons** • To record experience • To enhance personal ownership of learning • To engage in deep learning processes • To foster reflection and creative interaction in a group • To increase self-awareness and empowerment • To enhance creativity **Outcome reasons** • To learn from experience • To enhance other forms of learning • To understand personal learning processes • To enhance problem-solving skills • To develop the professional self in practice • For therapeutic and behaviour-changing purposes • To free up writing and the representation of learning • To provide an alternative 'voice' for self-expression • For assessment of formal learning

Style, form and contents derive from the main purposes of keeping a reflective journal and from the eventual involvement of someone as supervisor, 'reflective friend' or similar who can read it on a regular basis. For example, this tool has been shown to be very effective for students, especially when involved in their first experience of field practice. According to the people implicated and their roles, Jasper (2004) identifies:

- solitary journals (only one person is involved in writing and reading);
- 'writer–writes–reader-reads' journals (for example, students write and their practice teachers read to better guide the learning process);
- dialogue journal (it may be used in similar situations like the previous point, but here teachers interact with students also writing in the journal);
- group journals (social workers and other professions in teams may choose to enhance their common understanding, learning and reflection by tracking these processes in written form; many hands compose the content of the journal).

Journals can be more or less structured. Social workers may write whatever and however they want or they may react to given tasks and exercises, reply to specific questions and use a reflective framework, separate description from reflection in two different spaces (on the same page or on two different pages). Blogs and other similar sites published on the internet may be considered new forms of individual or collective reflective journals.

Among some of the techniques for structuring journals, Jasper (2004, p 109) mentions the focused topic areas journal, 'used where a specific topic is focused on in order to structure the learning to be achieved' and the project/research journals and diaries 'used specifically to keep an on-going reflective log of the progress of a project or research study'. The first of these two specific forms looks particularly interesting for the topic of this book and may suggest writing reflective journals focused only on mistakes. Nevertheless, a stimulating alternative may be represented by 'success journals', aimed at including descriptions of and reflection on unexpected achievement of desired professional goals and of attempted activities. This may lead to enhanced self-confidence that may be jeopardised by an excessive attention to failures from a negative perspective.

Lastly, it is interesting to note that some of the activities Moon (2006, pp 142–4) mentions as useful to encourage reflective writing in journals for personal development:

- take a theme (an object is chosen to focus attention and provide a starting point);
- use questions (like the ones from reflective frameworks);
- generate questions (learners are asked to develop their own questions);
- footprints ('on a particular topic, learners are asked to list around seven experiences [memories] of the topic in strict chronological order – from birth towards the present time');
- concept mapping or graphic representations of ideas ('concept map encapsulates an idea and the themes radiate from the main idea and subdivide hierarchically');
- free-flow writing ('good means of freeing the style and thoughts of writers is to let writing free-flow on a topic, not correcting or criticising it for a period of time [e.g. ten minutes]');
- 'take a sentence' (when one sentence is taken 'from your readings that sparked your interest and write on its meaning');
- reflecting on own writing (by using 'a double entry technique where one side of the page is for descriptive writing and the other is for further reflections on that writing').

Metaphors, art and imagination as catalyst for reflection

Imagination is a powerful catalyst for reflection. There are several forms of creative reflective writing as already listed: writing the unsent letter (or email), to a nominated other person, writing as a journalist, writing a fantasy story and so on are all strategies that make use of creativity, imagination and artistry to see things from a different perspective and make use of a way of thinking differently from rational reasoning alone. This section enlarges the view on this important area of where to find tools for professional development and considers metaphors and images as some of the best strategies for going deeper in reflection in social work as well as other areas. In fact, often the answers to the most important questions do not come rationally but rather intuitively and appear under the aspect of **metaphors** described in words or represented by pictures that can summarise objective and emotional components of an experience that may otherwise be indescribable. A metaphor is a 'compactor of communication', can express what is 'hard to express in literal language' and can 'capture the vividness of an experience' (McIntosh, 2010, pp 119–20).

The mental manipulation of images is important in any learning process because any metaphor conveys a holistic understanding of the action and so may bridge the gap between objectivity and subjectivity, between facts and values. This is well illustrated by the case of a social work student who, when he was doing his internship, described himself as an android, half man, half robot. This metaphor carries many aspects that would require several words to be fully described and is connected, among other things, to formal theories of organisational, sociological studies on professions, feelings of alienation and painful conflict of values between the intransigence imposed by bureaucratic procedures and values of respect for the individual (Gould, 1996).

This process of thought is not linear even if generally it goes through a series of steps that McIntosh (2010, pp 169–71) defines as follows:

1. reflective reproduction. It consists in the development of 'images' as data collections both 'self-generated and self-collected by the individuals who engage in the active imagination process';
2. immersion in reflective reproduction, when individuals immerse themselves within 'the developmental process of the forming of the reflective reproduction and the critical commentary';
3. establishing dialogical potential, between unconscious (where the reflective reproduction emerges from) and conscious levels;
4. establishing a transcendent potential. The ego stops its 'wish to dominate the decisions over what is and what is not relevant to the process'. What is not logical or coherent is acknowledged, bringing new and unexpected discoveries and findings;

5. hearing and orchestrating the reflective voices. Contradictory ideas and feelings may arise quite chaotically and the resulting situation could be like an orchestra playing without a conductor. It is important to let all these 'voices' move towards a harmonious synthesis;

6. reflexive emergence. A kind of 'illumination emerges out of the imagination and dialogic process which triggers an engagement in theoretical bodies of knowledge'.

In short, on one side imagination provides the informational base on which to apply the reflective thinking, on the other side metaphors and internal or even external dialogue lead to a deeper understanding of the experience and help to develop new actions.

How can social workers produce the literary or visual images mentioned earlier? One of the options, for example, is to ask **hypothetical questions**. They are commonly used by social workers during interviews with service users in order to help the users to enlarge their view on their lives and problems. Similarly this kind of question may be very productive if self-directed, like 'If your life right now was described by the image of a river, what would your river look like?' (Cheng, 2010, p 490). A river may be a metaphor for life, or for its professional aspect, and can give interesting insights. Similar results can be achieved by doing one of the following exercises proposed by Bolton (2010, p 45):

> The story of your work
> 1. If your work were a book, film, play or radio programme what would it be? A romantic, detective or fantasy novel, diary, roadmap or atlas, telephone directory, DIY (Do It Yourself) manual [...] reality television show [...]? [...]
> 2. Describe it.
> 3. Reread with positive imaginative insight, add or alter if you wish.

Other examples of creative exercises to reflect in depth on positive and negative aspects of situations are (Bolton, 2010, p 83):

Positive and negative
1. Write three sentences describing the sort of person you are (no one else need ever see this).
2. What characteristics do you think you excluded: be honest.
3. How many 'nots' are there (for example, I'm not good at numbers), compared to positives?
4. Rewrite these negatives as positives.
5. Reread and reflect positively.

Wild solutions
1. Describe a work problem, occasion, or person which puzzles you.
2. List your hunches about it: go on be wild.
3. Reread and choose one to write more about, thinking: What if ….
4. Reread with loving attention, altering as you wish.

The same author suggests an interesting method called 'Through the mirror' of reflective writing (Bolton, 2010, p 122–3):

1. Write for *six minutes* following the flow of your mind, as above, without stopping and without rereading till you've finished.
2. Follow-on writing: write for about 20 minutes about 'A Time in My Experience' as above. Remember this is for you. You need never share it with anyone, or without redrafting it first. Try to choose the first event which comes to mind, even if you have no idea why you have thought of it. Your writing will tell you why it is important. Trust it to do that.
3. Read all your writing to yourself, and alter or adapt as seems good. Are there any connections between the *six minutes'* write and the Follow-on? Note any reflections which occur to you as you read.

Any failure in professional life or any other kind of event may be chosen. While writing it is important to take the first event that comes to mind without any kind of judgement or fear that someone is going to read whatever will be on the paper (or on a computer file). A 'reflective friend' may be involved in the reflection on the material produced but it is better to take the decision on if and who to involve only after the act of writing is over.

Creative reflective writing has many forms, even play writing and acting (Rawal, 2009) and the use of **dreams** as a starting point to deepen the reflection, as described by Stimson (2009), who uses the Ullman experiential dream group as a tool in reflective practice for professionals and students. In this case, dreams are not treated as in psychotherapy or counselling but their descriptions are used to mobilise the intuitive sensitivity and creative unconscious in the people involved. For example, dreams, even if only partially remembered, can be continued in daytime as stories in written form or can be described as scripts of plays highlighting the main characters, events and stages of the narrative. Questions sometimes arise from dreams and these can be used to guide reflection on experiences in real professional life (Kaplan–Williams, 1980).

For many people it is easier to reflect in writing, but some practitioners prefer to **audio** record their reflection immediately after the event so as not to lose any benefits from the event. Then they listen to the recorded audio and go deeper in their reflection. Even **videoing** events like supervision meetings, interactions with peers or even the person him/herself talking in front of a camera can be a rich source of reflection (Ingram et al, 2014, p 27).

Words are important but **pictures and drawing** may lead deeper and turn out to be the most interesting source in many reflection processes. In fact, visual thinking may be exceptionally productive because images portray details and relationships that cannot be retyped in any verbal code and add new information to their corresponding logical-linguistic formulations. When words and abstract thinking do not allow us to solve a problem, the 'mind's eye' can help, using drawing images, diagrams or charts. Without any special preparation or competence everybody can use visual thinking as a strategy in a wide range of situations, from everyday life to professional or interpersonal problems and any activity of study (Antonietti et al, 1995). In fact, any abstract idea can be made concrete through drawing an image.

For example, as a powerful source of insight and personal development, Tate (2013) proposes drawing a tree, suspending any form of censure and self-judgement, or even take pictures of trees and choose one. This image can be explored from different angles and interrogated with questions like: What is it? What does it mean for me? How does this impact on me?

Drawings can be included in reflective journals or become the most important if not exclusive component of them. In this second case the result may consist in a prim and proper '**reflective visual journal**', that is 'a notebook with unlined pages in which individuals record their experiences using both imagery and written text' (Deaver and McAuliffe, 2009, p 615). 'As opposed to writing which is a linear process, drawing is more fluid and dynamic' so ideas and thoughts can 'be captured quickly and without formal attention to details, such as grammar or semantics' (Tokolahi, 2010, p 162).

Nevertheless, as Deaver and McAuliffe (2009, p 627) suggest, 'including responsive writing in the visual journaling process seemed to maximize the potential of art making'. So comments added to doodles, sketches or any other kind of image drawn and coloured using pens, pencils, crayons or similar are even better in making sense of experiences, especially the complex and the most emotionally intense ones. In fact, as Tokolahi (2010, p 168) says:

> [the] use of imagery and metaphors promotes abstract, non-linear thinking, enabling the person reflecting to access inner resourcefulness and unconscious processes, thus enhancing the reflective process and providing an alternative method for transforming learning and gaining insight. Given the ability to disguise issues in imagery, drawing-based journaling also provides a more confidential means of producing and transporting documented reflections in public arenas. Use of a drawing-based journal for

reflection is also noted to be useful as a strategy for stress reduction.

The best example of a mix of images and words is probably the so-called **mind maps**. What is a mind map and how to do it? Buzan (1996) suggests taking a blank sheet of white paper, writing the main concept at the centre of it and drawing lines to include any related concepts as shown in Figure 4.2, a mind map made by the author of this book to represent the structure of this chapter. Images, colours, different sizes and shapes, arrows and personal symbols emphasise, associate and clarify the concepts that are usually described with one word or a very few words. The more colours and pictures are used, the more significant the map is. Everybody may develop their own style. This tool is good to summarise and remember any kind of subject of study, but it may be used for creative purposes or to explore an event in depth as well. It is also a good support for memory since it combines visual with other mnemonic forms more related to abstract concepts and associations. Once created, maps can be modified anytime and/or visually explored to find new connections and meanings.

Figure 4.2: Mind map of chapter four

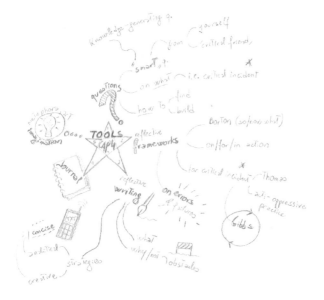

Chapter summary

1 Reflection and reflective practice may be considered at three levels: personal, dyadic (one-to-one) and with a multiplicity of people in groups or even in organisations. In all cases, 'smart questions' are the core of an effective reflection. 'Smart questions' puzzle, and lead search and thinking in new directions and into new areas.

2 A critical incident is 'any occurrence which was significant to a person for whatever reason' (Green Lister, 2012, p 108) and from which the professional wants to learn (Fook and Gardner, 2007). Reflection on critical incidents is highly productive especially if it is carried out using knowledge-generating questions.

3 Also 'critical friends' (who can offer external perspectives to extend your reflective capacity) and deficit-based and strength-based questions empower reflective practice.

4 Reflection is a process nurtured by questions. The quality of the latter determines the quality and depth of reflection. 'Smart questions' may be formulated by practitioners or these may use predefined questions, that is, reflective frameworks like Gibbs' reflective cycle and the reflective framework proposed in this chapter for an in-depth reflection on errors and failures.

5 Reflective writing is the deliberate use of strategies of writing as a way of reflecting and learning from experience. There are two types of reflective writing: analytical (characterised by objectivity and the attempt to stand back from the events considered) and creative (using imagination, metaphors and emotions, sometimes, in their rawest forms).

6 Strategies of concise reflective writing (that is, with a limited number of words, as in SMS and titles, for example) are very effective because they produce rich material that gives a global view on what happened and is not too much influenced by the final episodes and the moment when the reflection is carried out.

7 Any form of metaphor, written or drawn in a picture, may express the vibrancy of an experience and any related

emotions and feelings much better than only literal language. Audio and video recordings, mind maps and drawing in or out of visual reflective journals are some of the most effective reflective tools involving imagination and creativity.

FIVE

Feedback and other tools for learning together from mistakes in organisations

Learning outcomes

After this chapter you will be able to:

1 welcome any feedback from colleagues and service users as powerful resources of professional growth;
2 refine feedback from blame so as to highlight the helpful advice that is always in any feedback;
3 respond to feedback assertively;
4 identify and use conceptual tools to understand the complexity behind a 'bad' accident rather than look for a 'scapegoat';
5 use some tools that may help in changing practices and procedures when the latter have lost their original purpose.

Introduction

So far, learning from error has been seen as an activity people carry out through moments of reflection mostly in solitude or, in quite rare and lucky circumstances, with 'reflective friends'. However, social workers do not act alone but are included in networks of relationships with other professionals both inside and outside the organisations where they work. In addition, individual learning is part of a wider process producing organisational learning that is not the simple sum of what individuals know but includes the additional knowledge produced by exchanges and interactions between people.

This last chapter is focused on **tools and strategies** available in order to improve the quality of reflection and reflective practice **in cooperation with colleagues or the entire organisation** where social workers are employed. So the following pages are centred on some areas where reflection together with other people is especially fruitful: criticisms between colleagues and organisational processes like, for example, those involving risk management.

In every workplace there is a certain amount of criticism among colleagues and this is often seen more as a problem than an opportunity. In fact criticism is nothing more than a form of feedback, aimed at reporting an error made by one person to another, even if unfortunately it is seen more often as an unfavourable judgement on the whole person. What is felt as an attack often leads to a defence reaction that, on the other side, is seen as an aggression requiring a reaction and so a symmetric exchange of aggressive communication continues, leading, in some cases, to an escalation that is dangerous for the maintenance of peace in the workplace. In contrast, constructive criticism can help colleagues to see something that they were not able to see and be aware of because of their deep involvement in situations where the mistake was made.

In this chapter different types of **criticism** (relevant, unjustified, vague) are described and some assertive strategies for dealing with them are offered in order to help transform unjustified and vague criticism into something relevant and useful. The basic idea is to be aware of and distinguish the two different aspects, **content and relationship**, in every communicative interaction to be focused on the useful information coming from somebody else's perspective and to deal with the relationship in a more constructive way, so satisfying the universal needs of being recognised and appreciated. The assertive techniques described in this chapter can help to get the best from the criticism received, but they can also be used when a colleague does something wrong. In many cases and no matter how difficult and delicate it is, nobody can shirk the duty of reporting mistakes, first of all, to those who made them and for the greater good of the service users.

The second part of the chapter briefly presents some of the opportunities offered by **organisational management** processes dealing with quality and risk. In both cases the basic idea is rooted in a shared learning starting from a mistake, often defined as 'non-conformity' in many quality systems. What went wrong leads to meetings and discussions in order to minimise the harm produced and to implement processes for improving the organisation in those features that have been revealed as more fragile and at risk. These processes are activated only when organisational **procedures** are used as a means to an end, rather than an end in themselves. For example, filling in a form is done so as to have a better service, not to 'soil' a sheet of paper with a pen. If they are not working any longer, procedures have to be changed so they can serve their purpose and reason of existence once more: that is, the rights and wellbeing of service users.

What do you do when (you think) your colleague is wrong?

The focus of this section can be described in many ways and take many forms (criticism, blame, advice), but the more neutral term 'feedback' seems more appropriate to demonstrate how important evaluative responses from other people are in order to improve social workers' performances. These other people may be colleagues but also service users. In this last case, different kinds of positive effects have been discussed and demonstrated in many services, especially in health care organisations (Ghaye, 2008). Precious opportunities to develop services may arise through appropriate feedback and reflection upon it. Of course, feedback may be positive or negative but the more ideas for improvement there are, the more the benefits that come from them can involve practitioners who are keen to do better. For this reason, too, it is important to create systems of communication able to collect information on service users' points of view and suggestions.

Social workers are included in several networks inside and outside their organisations. Under certain conditions, if shared, their day-by-day learning may become organisational learning that is not a mere sum of the knowledge of individuals, but a process and product leading organisations to develop better strategies. People learn by reflecting on their experiences, successes and failures, but they also look at and reflect on what their colleagues do. They may keep their opinions to themselves or express them, for example, to those who have made some kind of mistake.

In a recent exploratory research study on the attitudes of health and social workers to their colleagues' mistakes, the two most important questions were: is it better to tell or not to tell colleagues they did something wrong? And, if you decide to tell them, how can this be done in an effective way (Sicora, 2010)? A widespread awareness of blindness to one's own mistakes is probably the strongest argument in favour of a positive answer to the first question. Telling colleagues about mistakes is a way of helping professional development but also a way to prevent bad consequences for service users and for social workers, who may pay dearly for their wrong moves. But it is often difficult to say "Hey, you are wrong!" and some practitioners confess they are able to do it only in a few grave cases. A good-quality relationship is the strongest facilitator, resulting, for example, from a history of mutual reports ("I always tell her and she always tells me when I am wrong"), a bad-quality relationship is the most important obstacle, as well as the fear of an angry reaction. Moreover, before saying something, people should double check before saying something in case they see what seems to be an error at first sight. Face-to-face talks in structured meetings in small or large groups were considered the best ways, according to the personal preferences of the social workers who were involved in the research.

Even if it is not always easy, the most fruitful way to be helped to do better at work is to listen to feedback coming from colleagues in the form of advice or criticisms (defined here as reports of error). Advice becomes actionable (and so 'good') when made in ways the human mind can turn into action coming from the embedded theories-in-use. These are what people really employ and they are often different from the espoused theory, which is what people say they are doing (Argyris, 2000).

When talking about the importance of feedback for practice teachers in social work, Doel et al (1996, p 79) refuse to use the adjectives 'positive' and 'negative' but prefer to use the words 'affirmative' and 'challenging' to highlight the essence of valuable sources of information. But it is true that not all kinds of feedback are equal. Hathaway (1990, pp 20–1) states that there are three **kinds of feedback**: '(1) Valid, bona fide, critical feedback, (2) unjustified, or invalid critical feedback, and (3) critical feedback that is vague or is simply a difference of opinion'. Positive answers to one or more of the following questions help in recognising whether feedback is valid:

- Do I hear the same feedback from more than one person?
- Does the critic know a great deal about the subject?
- Are the critic's standards known and reasonable?
- Is the critical feedback really about me? Or is the critic merely having a bad day or upset about something else?
- How important is it for me to respond to the critical feedback?

Vague feedback may need further exploration to extract any useful information that could be embedded in it. Some of the assertive techniques illustrated in this chapter may serve this purpose.

Nevertheless, before going further, it is important to bring the reader's attention to two of the core questions to reflect on when feedback arrives: What is the feedback saying about the relationship between the parties involved? What is it saying about the content?

Watzlawick et al (1967, p 52, emphasis added) affirm that **'every communication has a content and a relationship aspect** such that the latter classifies the former and is therefore a meta-communication'. "This is an order" and "I'm just kidding" are examples of meta-communication and define the nature of the relationship between the two parties involved (exercise of power or manifestation of friendship).

If someone stops and asks a stranger for directions in a street ("Where can I find the closest restaurant?"), the latter can give the same information (for example, "Go straight ahead, then turn left and then right"), but using a very annoyed tone of voice so as to communicate without using words, the message "You are a nuisance," or he may say exactly the same thing but with a gentle voice and with a smile, thus showing a welcoming attitude. These are dynamics that occur frequently in social work as well. Feedback, in fact, has a strong relational component and many problems arise from the fact that people are not aware of this. People defend and attack when they receive feedback perceived as 'negative'; they lose sight of the content of the communication and are more focused on relationship messages perceived as "You are a menace, an enemy." Instead, focusing on the content can eliminate the 'poison' from the feedback and prevent an escalation of reciprocal blame and conflicts.

What has all of this to do with feedback or, more precisely, with feedback on mistakes? There is a lot to learn and apply since public perception of the goal may be very different from the intended outcome, and evident intentions may be different from hidden and even unconscious ones. What are people verbally or non-verbally saying when they say "You are wrong"? Is what they are saying and what the other side hears: "You made a mistake" or rather "You are a mistake"? Or "I value you and your skills for growing professionally or personally" or "I want to show how incompetent you are (and how skilled I am)"?

These dynamics are essential to understanding the nature of the main **obstacles** to soliciting, accepting and incorporating feedback in social work practice. Previously, in chapter two, one of the biases mentioned for its relevance to the topic of this book was called 'wariness of lurking conflict', occurring when 'staff may be anxious in case they are assaulted, [the] subject of complaints, sued, censured, criticised by inquiries, the media or politicians, etc.' (Taylor, 2013, p 70).

Brown (2012) highlights a connection between shame, including the shame of being wrong, and vulnerability, since the first may convince people they are not good, competent or professional enough and stop them 'daring' to be creative and innovative because of the fear of being criticised. In contrast, 'shame resilience' may help to fight against 'shame-prone cultures', where people are encouraged to connect their self-worth to what they produce rather than what they are. When it becomes fear, shame leads to risk aversion and to the death of any innovation, which, in social work, can mean it becomes impossible to help service users when they are stuck in hard and unprecedented problems.

Giving advice is not difficult, but, as also highlighted in the research mentioned at the beginning of this section, it is harder and more difficult to criticise someone because it is often very troublesome to admit a mistake. This tendency is rooted in cognitive dissonance and is so strong and common that even false memories may be built for self-justification in the attempt to protect low self-esteem. This may occur with the most unexpected people: celebrities, powerful politicians, men or women of state and others who seem very self-confident. These efforts at finding excuses to justify being wrong are designed to serve the very human need all people have to feel good about what they have done, what they believe, and who they are. Yet at all ages people can learn to see that mistakes are not so terrible but are inevitable and help everybody to grow and become better (Tavris and Aronson, 2007).

Nevertheless, **'blame culture'** is pervasive in any organisation. Taylor (2013, p 156) suggests reflecting on the following questions to gain more awareness of this issue and its connection with decision making in social work and risk of mistakes producing bad consequences for service users:

- Do you feel you are working in a 'blame culture'?
- What are the main sources of pressure that you think would influence you to feel 'blamed' if a tragedy ensued after a decision?
- What do you think are appropriate mechanisms for accountability of professional and organisational decision making in your ideal society?
- What might be done by the social work profession to support you more in professional judgements and decision making?
- What might be done by your employer to support you more in judgements and decision making?
- What might you do so that if a tragedy were to ensure, your judgements and decision-making processes would still be regarded as sound?

Moving away from a blame culture is possible if the will to do so is authentic and helped by a good use of appropriate messages of relationship, expressing appreciation and trust in the other people. Table 5.1 provides some examples on how the same sentence can be said in two different forms of culture. It is important to be aware of how much is said in terms of relationship when people give feedback and that a slightly different tone of voice or context may dramatically turn the meaning of the sentence from "You are worthless and incompetent" to "You are valuable and competent."

Table 5.1: From blame to appreciation (Ghaye, 2008, p 124)

Statement	Blame culture	Statement culture
"You will do better next time"	Threat	Encouragement
"I didn't expect you to do it that way"	Reprimand	Opinion
"You need to take a break"	Order	Concern
"I haven't seen it done like that before"	Contempt	Interest
"Well that's certainly a different approach to tackling the problem"	Sarcasm	Observation
"Let's wait and see, shall we?"	Dismissive	Curiosity
"Why have you done it like that?"	Accusation	Enquiry
"I know what to do"	Control	Reassurance
"It would certainly help if you read up on that"	Frustration	Invitation
"Just watch me, I'll show you how to do it"	Annoyance	Demonstration

Skills to turn from the first meaning to the second meaning in Table 5.1 may be developed and strengthened, and could be listed as integrity, concern for the others, awareness of the worth of differences, desire to help others to develop, optimism, ability to stretch goals and aptitude to listen (Folkman, 2006).

Giving and receiving feedback assertively

How to get the most from feedback? Some assertive techniques may help to strengthen collaborative relationships between colleagues and offer opportunities for professional development by learning from mistakes.

Doel et al (1996) describe some steps in receiving feedback that are designed for social work practice teaching but may also be useful for experienced practitioners who want to grow by reflecting together in pairs or in a team. First, it is important to be aware of any personal response in receiving feedback, defensive or even aggressive reactions included. Then proactive attitudes in terms of asking for feedback may help and increase the quantity and quality of any valuable source of information from other people. Finally, when unfair comments are received and could produce frustration, especially on days when feelings of vulnerability are stronger, it is useful not to deny the other people's perceptions but to let them know that there could be different opinions on the same issues. In this case, when feedback is too unpleasant, it is much better to postpone any further evaluation, just saying that a better moment will be found to consider and use it to influence practice positively.

Smith (1975) identifies three **strategies to face manipulative criticisms** or, using the typology described in the previous section, unjustified or vague feedback and 'separate' the truth ("You forgot to call the service users") from the arbitrary ("A good practitioner never forgets to call service users"): fogging, negative assertion and negative inquiry. They reduce the potentially negative content in feedback, improve the quality of the listening and reduce risks of symmetric escalations.

The first (fogging) consists in not denying the received criticism and not reacting with parallel blame. Metaphorically the respondent has to be like a 'fog bank', which does not allow people to clearly see through it. In this case, when replying, it is possible to agree with: (1) any truth (agreeing with truth) or (2) any possible truth in statements (agreeing with the odds) or (3) with the general truth in logical statements (agreeing in principle) people use to criticise. The following examples in a case of the late delivery of a report clarify these three possibilities:

- Statement from A: "You presented me your last report after the deadline I gave you." Assertive reply from B: "That is true. I was late in giving you my last report."
- Statement from A: "If you are so often late you can damage our entire organisation." Assertive reply from B: "You could be right." (Or, "I agree with you. If I were not late I would probably make a better contribution to our organisation").
- Statement from A: "You know how important being efficient is to any social worker. If you keep being late so often, you won't look like a good practitioner. You do not want that to happen, do you?" Assertive reply from B: "You are right. What you say makes sense, so when I want to make a better impression, I will give my report in earlier."

Negative assertion is a second strategy to keep respect and self-respect and, at the same time, cope with mistakes with the sincere intention to learn from them. This happens when people assertively accept what is wrong in their behaviour saying, for example, "I gave you my report the day after the deadline." This sentence may prevent an escalation of charges and counter-charges.

Finally (the previous two may be combined with this last strategy), 'negative inquiry' is aimed at requesting specific feedback and forcing the critics to look at potential solutions, especially when they have given vague or unjust feedback. For example, "This report is not accurate" is quite vague and useless in guiding the other towards its improvement. A reply like "I don't understand. What is it about my report that is bad?" is an assertive response aimed at better understanding what is wrong so as to collect suggestions in order to correct and write a better report. "What, specifically, did I do wrong that …", "If you were me, what would you do differently?", "I'm not sure I fully understand what you mean, could you please give me some examples …" are all good starting points to build a 'negative inquiry' that gives a positive relational message ("I value you and your skills to give me good suggestions") and allows the person to collect detailed information on how to correct a mistake.

A similar attention to relationships is essential too, when people are told they are wrong. So **what is the best way to give constructive feedback**? Again, it is important to be fully aware of the two levels of communication and to be positive in terms of relational message. There are many 'elegant' approaches (that is, approaches without any element of attack), like the 'sandwich' one, when the criticism is between two slices of tasty compliments: "I think you did a very good job. It would be perfect if only you could … [here there is the major criticism]. But, overall, as I told you, you did a great job" (Harford, 2011).

The Describe, Acknowledge, Specify, Reaffirm (DASR) script is one of the best techniques in taking feedback out of the blame culture and into the statement one. Hathaway (1990, pp 51–2) describes its four steps as follows:

- DESCRIBE what you observed in terms of behaviour. Use factual information. Use sensory language – what you saw, counted, touched, smelled, heard. Use statistical information relative to quantity, frequency, duration, size.

  'When you …', 'I saw this happen …', 'The reports indicate the following …'

  Vague information is rarely useful. If you have 'sensed' something is happening, however, you may with many thorough discussions with others, be able to be more specific. Consider how you can provide specific evidence or examples of performance. Analyse the pros and cons of the words and phrases you use to give feedback.

- ACKNOWLEDGE your reactions to what happened or the impact of the behaviour. Think first about what you are trying to achieve (the outcome desired) and what you wish to say. Concentrate on expressing ideas and reactions as clearly, sincerely, and concisely as possible. Use simple and responsive language.

'I feel unsure, frustrated, concerned about ...' 'I disagree with what you did because ...'

'The impact on the team is ...'

Aim for consistency between what you say and how you say it. Keep in mind your goal of increased understanding and a change in the other person's behaviour.

- SPECIFY. Ask explicitly for a different, specified behaviour. The language you use here can be instrumental in either building motivation or undermining the person's enthusiasm. Say 'What I would prefer ...'

- REAFFIRM their worth and ability to correct their behaviour. Say, perhaps, 'I have confidence that you can do the job correctly.'

Adapting one of the examples given by the same author (Hathaway, 1990, p 58), a manager in a rest house could try and build an assertive feedback to address two workers who talk more to each other than to the service users this way:

'Mrs. John and Mrs. Smith, I am concerned that our users are feeling ignored because you are talking to each other rather than to them when they called you some minutes ago. I'd prefer that you talk with them when requested so as to make them feel more comfortable. I feel confident that doing so will help to make our job better and more satisfying for all.'

Of course, in this and in any other case it is important to be clear about the purpose in giving feedback. An authentic attempt to contribute to learning from past failures and mistakes may be effective only when there is trust in the honest intention and capability of the other party. If there is mistrust or lack of confidence in the other party, an assertive strategy may be useless, if not counterproductive, and lead to conflict in the workplace.

Reflection in groups

'Reflective friends' and feedback from colleagues and service users lead individuals to enrich the level of their learning noticeably, including when they reflect on their mistakes. The outcome of two or more people reflecting is much more than the simple sum of the individual acquiring awareness and professional skills.

Several authors have highlighted the importance of reflecting in groups in health and social services. According to Carter (2013), groups for reflection or peer supervision are aimed at developing the capability and the competence of their participants; they have particular benefits and risks but also specific challenges. They are especially suitable for developing new ideas, providing an apt environment for creativity and peer support, learning from others and giving the opportunity for superior insight thanks to the heterogeneity of the participants. At the same time, as in any group, they can make some members feel uncomfortable or there could be some abuse of power. In that case, when talking about their experiences, failures and mistakes, some people could feel too exposed and vulnerable. Good **facilitators** may help these groups to obtain better results when they skilfully manage group dynamics, starting from expressing clear, explicit and shared aims and by using time appropriately and protecting confidentiality. Any meeting, but especially the first, has to be prepared carefully and conducted accordingly. Before the meeting, it is important to find a venue, decide an appropriate and sufficient time, invite the people and inform them about the aims of the group. At the start of the first meeting 'ice breakers' may be appropriate to help participants get to know each other. Then it is also useful to inform the participants that listening, being non-judgemental, having the right to stay silent are ground rules and, even though it may happen that someone feels uncomfortable at times, everything will be done to deal with this and reach the maximum possible comfort at the end. The participants may be encouraged to recall events they want to discuss using the chosen reflective framework. Notes can be taken and may help to summarise at the end when it is good to check whether the participants feel okay or if there is any reason for dissatisfaction or discomfort.

Fook and Gardner (2007) have developed a model for critical reflection in small groups, providing theory and a detailed description of the process, which is structured in two main stages: the first is aimed at expressing the fundamental assumptions that are implicit in the descriptions of the participants' experience; the second is focused on how practice can be improved by the new and deeper awareness that has been gained in the first stage. Here too the group facilitator is essential to bring about the best outcome of the whole process.

Furthermore, leadership is essential in any kind of collaborative working, including when reflective practice is involved. Since sharing deeper understandings and, sometimes, unexpected insights benefits any professional practice, transformational leadership should facilitate any process to create the conditions to release potential in the team (McCray, 2013).

Another collective situation that may develop learning from experience is **group supervision**. This is defined by Bond and Holland (1998, cited by Rolfe et al, 2001, p 101) as 'three or more people who come together and interrelate cooperatively with each other toward their common purpose of giving and receiving clinical supervision'. This form of group is becoming more popular as a consequence of a growing lack of resources for individual supervision, but is very different from that and is not merely supervision with an audience. An appropriate guide is important, since lack of proper facilitation may lead to the premature end of the group.

Finally, the combination of reflection in groups and reflective writing produces the '**collaborative multi-professional journal**' (Moon, 2006, p 79, emphasis added) where topics are 'practice-related learning, professional philosophies, personal learning and growth and reflective practice', and whose purposes are 'to connect with the others involved, to pose questions, the discussion of issues, the sharing of learning and capturing of stories'. This tool is useful for keeping track of the collective learning journey of a multi- or mono-professional team. Each practitioner writes in this journal and contributes to building a richer picture and understanding of the common experience by sharing different views and perspectives.

Reflection in a group, in meetings and/or with collaborative journals may not only empower individual learning considerably but also provide very instructive lessons to a group of practitioners in the same organisations or even in different organisations, starting from a case study proposed by a member of the group. Even if the pressure to work efficiently is strong and less time and fewer resources are left for continuous training, supervision and other forms of structured reflection, meeting in a group to reflect on a mistake one or more members have experienced would be of great benefit for the entire team and organisation. Giving some structure and rules is essential, as is choosing appropriate reflective frameworks (from the many proposed in this book) to guide the discussion. One meeting of approximately 90 minutes (or more, if possible) a month, or even less frequently, may provide unexpected fruitful results, thus improving the quality of social work services given to service users.

Reflective organisations and mistakes

Individuals, pairs, groups and organisations seem like steps in increasing complexity. However, individuals have to consider the role of organisations and vice versa. Thinking about social work practice, it is easy to recognise that there is never one simple cause of any occurrence in the intricate systems the practitioners meet daily. If there is not only one cause, there is not even one person to blame if something went wrong. It is not single elements but entire systems and their interactions that are 'responsible' for failures and mistakes. This is not an attempt to avoid making someone feel responsible (and responsibility is different from guilt) when his or her role in any harm is relevant, it is a way to consider the whole problem in its complexity, to learn from experience and to act in order to avoid similar mistakes in the future. As highlighted in the first two sections of this chapter, if someone does something wrong, it is much better to give useful feedback than to lay unfruitful blame.

The so-called '**Swiss cheese model**' described by Reason (1990) provides a very good description for considering the cause of accidents, not only in technological systems but also in any other kind of complex system. There are basic elements in any type of production, in case of services too, not only for goods, and they can be represented as layers, one behind the other (in brackets some possible application in the social work context has been added to Reason's model):

1 decision makers (policy makers, etc.),
2 line management (related to operations, maintenance, training and, in general, implementation of the strategies defined at the previous level 1);
3 preconditions (skills, knowledge, attitudes and motivations of any workers involved in the process, environmental conditions, codes of practice, physical and psychological conditions, etc.);
4 productive activities (what happens in the 'here and now' of the specific social work intervention);
5 defences (any safeguards against foreseeable hazards like, for example, an alarm system to activate in case of risk of aggression, or a colleague reading and double-checking a report before sending it to the authority who has to decide on sensitive cases).

As shown in Figure 5.1, any of these layers may have one or more 'holes', which represent fallible decisions, deficiencies or unsafe acts. As Reason (2000, p 769) says:

> in an ideal world each defensive layer would be intact. In reality, however, they are more like slices of Swiss cheese, having many holes — though unlike in the cheese, these holes are continually opening, shutting, and shifting their location. The presence of holes in any one 'slice' does not normally cause a bad outcome. Usually, this can happen only when the holes in many layers momentarily line up to permit a trajectory of accident opportunity — bringing hazards into damaging contact with victims.

Figure 5.1: Reason's Swiss Cheese Model

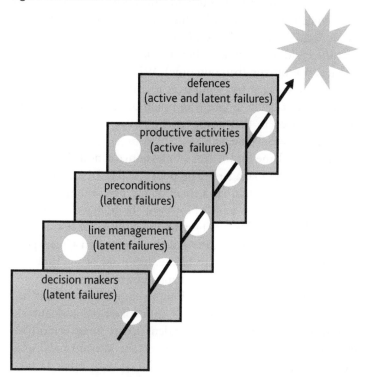

Source: Adapted from Reason, 1990.

A hypothetical (but maybe not too far from some realities) example could be thought of in the field of child protection. Policy makers in a period of economic crisis could decide to reduce the general expenditure for social welfare (decision makers). Consequently, the management of an important agency for child protection in a rural area declares there is no money to replace social workers who have retired. The managers of that agency instruct social workers to see children and their families exclusively in their offices because the workforce is reduced and consequently there is not so much time to visit these people at home (line management). The social worker Mary, who is young and not so experienced, meets a couple and their 4-year-old daughter at the end of a very intense and tiring day of work (precondition). Nothing worrying emerges during this interview, as she writes in her report (productive activities) and all her experienced colleagues are too busy working on their cases to help Mary to examine the situation in detail (defences). Some weeks later, a relative of the couple report to the police that the child was beaten by her drunk father so badly that her left arm was broken (bad outcome). When the police enter the house they see that the child lives in a dirty and unsafe room while the rest of the house is in much better condition. Mary has never been in that house so she has not noticed such an evident indicator of neglect.

Who is to blame for the lack of preventive action? Mary? Her colleagues? The managers? The policy makers? None of them and all of them. Each has a small or big part of responsibility but none has all the 'guilt'. Not even the policy makers who had to solve the problem of how to distribute fewer resources to different areas of activities. It would be easy to find a 'scapegoat' and personal inadequacies to blame, but most of the time this would not avoid bad accidents happening again.

Of course, situations are much more complex than described in this story, and in reality too root causes of serious accidents are mostly present long before the accident occurs. Some errors have evident effects immediately; some others are dormant and display their consequences only when combined with other factors. Detecting these latent errors is vital in order to prevent any kind of failure and harm. This may happen when the different layers described before are able to communicate and send each other feedback on what they can see from their peculiar point of view (Reason, 1990).

Blame is not at home in a **reflective organisation**, which is much more than the total sum of all practitioners reflecting because it includes any communication and feedback aimed both at understanding in depth, rather than blaming, and at improving services for users more than anything else. The preconditions for building such an organisation are sharing knowledge and vision, cognitive and organisational flexibility and challenging reflection within meetings with other social workers, but also two of the main focuses of this book: that is, learning from mistakes and asking for feedback (Ingram et al., 2014). Table 5.2 shows a grid to evaluate how reflective an organisation is.

Table 5.2: Grid to evaluate 'How reflective is my organisation?'

Settings	Open discussion	Sharing knowledge	Sharing vision	Acknowledge-ment of mistakes and lessons learned	Challenging and debating	Flexibility in thinking and systems	Opportunities to discuss personal values	Responsive	Acceptance of risks and uncertainty
Communication with • service users • peers • other professionals									
Meeting • service users • peers • other professionals									
Assessment									
Intervention									
Decision making									
Support and supervision									
Records and case notes									

Rating: 1 to 5, with 1 being not evident at all and 5 being very evident
Source: Ingram et al, 2014, p 157.

There are two diverse concepts close to, but different from the idea of reflective organisations: organisational learning and learning organisations. The first consists of any 'process through which learning takes place'; the second includes the 'characteristics of an organisation that learns'. The latter is favoured by systemic thinking, teamwork and work-based learning, but is hindered by any excessive attention to increase productivity and profit in a context of increased pressure of social services towards logics from market and commercial enterprises (Gould, 2004, pp 7, 2).

In this context leaders have to be reflective, that is they have to be brave, 'wise' (and not only skilled, clever and smart, according to widespread popular opinion), authentic and able to express their personality fully, to listen and to be open to others' opinions (Vitullo, 2006). Moreover, as already mentioned in chapter three (in the first section, 'Why do social workers "need" mistakes'), being open and democratic is not only a central attitude of any reflective leader but, together with the acceptance of the likelihood of error and the reliance on verifiable data, it is one of the three qualities of any successful **organisational error-prevention system** (Schulz, 2010).

Furthermore, in reflective organisations workers may express their dissent and managers allow dissent as the only way to change and adapt to the transformations of the environment. All organisations need rules but they are just means to achieve the organisational mission, which, in the case of social work, is the wellbeing of the users. When this is forgotten, rules and procedures become the main reason for the workers' activity, with paradoxical effects which may lead to a dramatic decrease in the quality of the services. On the other hand, actions that are effective in helping users may be considered 'deviant' and 'wrong' according to the organisational rules. In order to avoid this result it is important that health and social workers stand up and work to change their organisations and bring them back on track by giving appropriate feedback after an in-depth reflection on the procedures that seem to have lost their original purpose.

Taylor (2010, pp 113–15) proposes a framework designed for health care, but which may be used in social work services too. In the following questions 'procedure X' is a practice or procedure that has been established for some time but the value of which has now been called into doubt. The questions are divided into three sections:

- assessing and planning: an initial assessment of the problem and a plan for the development of an argument are made to set up the premises for rational thinking;
- implementing: an argument is developed by analysing the issues and assumptions operating in the situation;
- evaluating: the problem is reviewed using all the information obtained through the process of technical reflection.

At the end of this process, the hypothesis (the practice or procedure has lost its functionality or not) is either confirmed or disconfirmed in a succinct statement.

The complete list of the questions is presented in Table 5.3, because of its usefulness in social and health organisations and its relevance to the topic of this chapter.

Table 5.3: Framework to evaluate practices or procedures that seem to have lost their original functionality (adapted from Taylor, 2010, pp 113–15)

A. Assessing and planning
What is Procedure X?
Why is Procedure X done?
How is Procedure X done?
When is Procedure X done?
What are the outcomes of Procedure X?
Why do you believe that Procedure X is of questionable value? How do you propose to amend Procedure X?
What words and language are commonly associated with Procedure X?
Why are certain words and language commonly associated with Procedure X?
Is there any evidence of misuse of words and language in Procedure X?
Could the words and language commonly associated with Procedure X be stated differently?
What health care problems are associated with Procedure X?

B. Implementing
What arguments are made to support the continuation of Procedure X in its present form?
What health care assumptions underlie the support of Procedure X in its present form?
What premises support the argument for Procedure X in its present form?
Do these premises follow logically to provide sound conclusions?
If not, why not?
What inferences have been made and in what ways are they plausible in supporting Procedure X in its present form?
What arguments are made to support the discontinuation of Procedure X in its present form?
What health care assumptions underlie the opposition to Procedure X in its present form?
On what premises are these arguments for opposing Procedure X in its present form based?
Do these premises follow logically to provide sound conclusions?
If not, why not?
What inferences have been made and in what ways are they plausible in opposing Procedure X in its present form?

C. Evaluating
What information has been gained to date through implementing the technical reflection process?   In what ways can you verify, corroborate and justify claims, beliefs, conclusions, decisions and actions taken in this process?   What are the reasons for your beliefs and conclusions regarding this issue? What are your value judgements about this issue?   To what extent can you claim that the conclusions you have reached are sound? What other possible consequences may transpire due to the conclusions reached by this process?

Because of its many questions, this complex framework might require a lot of time to be fully applied, but it may guide collective and detailed reflections very effectively in order to understand if and why organisational procedures are off track and no longer serve their original purpose. Organisations are complex mechanisms aimed at goals that individuals cannot reach by themselves as single persons. Only collective reflections can lead to collective actions and then to organisational and social transformations. Working for social change to fight against marginalisation, social exclusion and oppression, and for social stability when it is not used to marginalise, exclude or oppress any particular group of persons, are essential parts of the core mandate of social work (IFSW and IASSW, 2014). Their realisation can be made step-by-step, starting from individual reflections but the involvement of groups and organisations is essential for any lasting and deep results.

Chapter summary

1. Blame culture is the main obstacle to expressing and listening to affirmative and useful feedback on mistakes.
2. Feedback is effective in helping professional development only if it is clear in its content and positive in terms of the message regarding the relationship between the giver and receiver of feedback.
3. Fogging, negative assertion and negative inquiry are useful assertive strategies in dealing with critical feedback. They reduce the potentially negative content in any feedback,

improve the quality of the listening and reduce risks of symmetric escalations.

4 The Describe, Acknowledge, Specify, Reaffirm (DASR) script is one of the best techniques for getting feedback out from the blame culture.

5 Reason's Swiss cheese model helps us to understand that any failure or 'bad' accident is produced by a combination of latent failures (these are not evident immediately) in the basic elements common to any social work system (decision makers, line management, preconditions, productive activities, defences).

6 A reflective organisation is much more than the total sum of all practitioners reflecting. It also includes any communication and feedback aimed at improving services for users.

7 Open and democratic communication, acceptance of the likelihood of error and reliance on verifiable data are central principles of any organisational error-prevention system.

8 Practices or procedures that have been established for some time may lose their capability to function properly as a consequence of changes in the environment. What is considered a mistake, according to that rule, may be the right thing to do to keep the focus on the wellbeing of service users. Reflection helps to change procedures and social work organisations and bring them back on track for their mission.

Conclusion:
The start of a never-ending process

From the reflective journal of the author of this book:

'**February 21st**. This morning I received an email from a student of mine asking whether the mark I had already registered and signed in the university system was correct or I considered the result of the exam she sat 17 days before but not the paper she sent me in December. I double-checked and she was right: I gave her 26 instead of 27, that is closer to the maximum of 30. I was upset: how did I make such a silly mistake? I am working hard and always try not to make any mistake that can damage my students. By the way, two weeks before the registration I wrote a notice on my bulletin board and asked the students to write to me within 5 days if they did not accept their mark. In that notice there was also the list of the students who had sent me the paper above and whom I had to add one mark to. But I did not include her name in the list by mistake! Why did she not tell me before? I heard that the procedure to correct it is complicated and I have to involve even the Rector.

'I hate to show my mistakes, especially to the Department Secretary who is always so strict with the teaching staff. I have even thought to write back to the student that I had already added the additional mark and that the correct sum is 26 or that I cannot make any change because she did not write to me before and the rules of our university do not allow any change now. The more I think about it the angrier

189

I get with myself also because I am angry for myself being unable to accept my error that, after all, is a small thing compared, for example, to what surgeons can make in operating rooms. Am I getting paranoid? I read so much on mistakes and am even writing a book on this topic! It is like I want the golden rule 'everybody makes mistakes' to apply to others but not to myself. I don't practise what I preach.

'I stop and reflect. Why do I have this excessive reaction? Do I really think that reflecting on mistakes will bring me to the 'lost paradise' of perfection? Why do I need to be considered perfect? Maybe I was wrong: reflection on mistakes does not make people perfect but just helps them to correct themselves and learn something new. It is impossible not to make mistakes but it is possible to correct them quicker and more effectively without any drama. But first of all I have to be aware of my mistakes and act accordingly. No need to be angry. Enjoy and learn from this experience.

'*February 22nd.* I wrote to the student that she is right and I am sorry for my mistake. I promised I will do my best to rectify her mark even if the procedure is not easy. I will keep her updated. I also asked her for some suggestions on how to write the notice in a more effective way so students can report any mistake to me more easily.

'In the meanwhile I called the Administration and received the information I asked for: the procedure to correct the mistake is easier and quicker than I expected. The person on the phone was very kind and told me what I too often forget, that is everybody (and, I add, I am not an exception) can make mistakes.

'*February 29th.* The mark has been officially rectified. In the past days the student wrote to me and thanked me for my prompt reaction and attention to her request. She is aware she would have had to

write to me before and does not have any advice on
how I can act differently.'

What will happen after reading this book and applying its
suggestions? Will readers make fewer mistakes? Probably not.
Will they have less unpleasant feelings when they are wrong?
Maybe yes, maybe no. Will their service users benefit from more
reflective social workers? Hopefully yes. And this yes is the reason
why this book was written.

After reflecting on the basic underlying concepts and using
the tools proposed in the previous pages, it will be easier and
take less time to **recognise** when mistakes are made ('mistakes
are inevitable and this does not mean I am a bad social worker,
neither that I am a victim of circumstances because others are
guilty and I have no responsibility for what happened'), to **reflect**
on what happened, to start working to **repair** any damage and
to keep the consequent **learning** ready for any similar occasion
in the future.

Getting rid of shame and guilty feelings does not give any
licence to be irresponsible, but, on the contrary, can significantly
improve any learning from mistakes because it makes it much
easier to **reflect with other people**. Social work is a tough
profession and working alone makes it even tougher. Together,
social workers can reflect, improve their skills and abilities, fight
against a useless 'blame culture' and, instead, build learning
organisations that never forget they exist to help people
not as an end in themselves. As mentioned in the previous
pages, acceptance of the likelihood of error and democratic
communication are two of the most important features of any
organisational error-prevention system (Schulz, 2010).

The **obsession with perfection** has a cost that is much
higher than that of paying reasonable attention to reduce mistakes
because people are human (imperfect but still the best thing that
everybody can be) and have limited resources. Time is limited
and excessive double-checking risks blocking other essential
activities and creates more risks and dangers.

It is clear that doing all this is not easy at all and failures in
learning from mistakes in social work are always around the
corner. Nevertheless, step-by-step this challenging adventure

may give more energy and inspiration to social workers, and make them more and more able to 'promote social change and development, social cohesion, and the empowerment and liberation of people' (IFSW and IASSW, 2014).

References

Abercrombie, N., Hill, S., Turner, B.S. (2006) *Dictionary of sociology* (5th edn), London: Penguin.

American Heritage® dictionary of the English language (5th edn), Boston, MA: Houghton Mifflin Harcourt, https://www.ahdictionary.com.

Antonietti, A., Angelini, C. and Cerana, P. (1995) *L'intuizione visiva: Utilizzare le immagini per analizzare e risolvere i problemi [Visual intuition: Using pictures to analyse and solve problems]*, Milano: FrancoAngeli.

Arendt, H. (1971) *Life of the mind*, vol. I: *Thinking*, San Diego: Harcourt Brace Jovanovich.

Argyris, C. (2000) *Flawed advice and the management trap*, Oxford: Oxford University Press.

Ash, A. (2013) 'A cognitive mask? Camouflaging dilemmas in street-level policy implementation to safeguard older people from abuse', *British Journal of Social Work*, 43(1): 99–115.

Association Nationale des Assistants de Service Social (ANAS) (1994) 'Code de déontologie', Paris, ifsw.org/publications/national-codes-of-ethics/france/.

Australian Association of Social Workers (2010) 'Code of ethics', Canberra, www.aasw.asn.au/document/item/1201.

AvenirSocial (2006) 'Codice deontologico degli operatori sociali', Berna, www.avenirsocial.ch/cm_data/CodiceDeontologico_A4_i.pdf.

Baldwin, M. (2004) 'Critical reflection: opportunities and threats to professional learning and service development in social work organizations', in N. Gould and M. Baldwin (eds) *Social work, critical reflection and the learning organization*, Aldershot: Ashgate, pp 41–55.

Bolton, G. (2010) *Reflective practice: Writing and professional development* (3rd edn), London: Sage.

Bond, M. and Holland, S. (1998) *Skills of clinical supervision for nurses*, Buckingham: Open University Press.

Borges, J.L. (1962) *Ficciones*, New York: Grove Press.

Borton, T. (1970) *Reach, touch and teach*, New York: McGraw-Hill.

Bradshaw, J. (1988) *Healing the shame that binds you*, Deerfield Beach, FL: Health Communications.

Brandon, M., Sidebotham, P., Bailey, S., Belderson, P., Hawley, C., Ellis, C. et al. (2012) *New Learning from serious case reviews: A two-year report for 2009–2011*. London: Department for Education.

Braye, S. and Preston-Shoot, M. (2016) *Practising social work law* (4th edn), Basingstoke: Palgrave Macmillan.

Braye, S., Orr, D. and Preston-Shoot, M. (2015a) 'Learning lessons about self-neglect? An analysis of serious case reviews', *Journal of Adult Protection*, 17(1): 3–18.

Braye, S., Orr, D. and Preston-Shoot, M. (2015b) 'Serious case review findings on the challenges of self-neglect: indicators for good practice', *Journal of Adult Protection*, 17(2): 75–87.

Brookfield, S. (1987) *Developing critical thinkers*, Buckingham: Open University Press.

Brown, R. (2012) *Daring greatly: How the courage to be vulnerable transforms the way we live, love, parent and lead*, New York: Gotham Books.

Brown, K. and Rutter, L. (2008) *Critical thinking for social work*, London: Sage.

Bruce, l. (2013) *Reflective practice for social workers: A handbook for developing professional confidence*, Maidenhead: Open University Press.

Bryans, P. (1999) 'What do professional men and women learn from making mistakes at work?' *Research in Post-Compulsory Education*, 4(2): 83–194.

Bulman, C. (2004) 'An introduction to reflection', in C. Bulman and S. Schutz (eds) *Reflective practice in nursing* (3rd edn), London: Blackwell, pp 1–24.

Bulman, C. and Schutz, S. (eds) (2013) *Reflective practice in nursing* (5th edn), London: Blackwell.

Butler, G. (2013) 'Reflection on emotions in social work', in C. Knott and T. Scragg (eds) *Reflective practice in social work* (3rd edn), London: Sage, pp 34–50.

Buzan, T. (1996) *The mind map book*, New York: Penguin.

Campanini, A. (2007) *L'intervento sistemico: Un modello operativo per il servizio sociale [The systemic intervention: An operating model for social work]*, Roma: Carocci.

Canadian Association of Social Workers (CASW) (2005a) 'Code of ethics', casw-acts.ca/sites/default/files/attachements/CASW_Code%20of%20Ethics.pdf.

Canadian Association of Social Workers (CASW) (2005b) 'Guidelines for ethical practice', casw-acts.ca/sites/default/files/attachements/CASW_Guidelines%20for%20Ethical%20Practice.pdf.

Canavan, J. (2006) 'Family Support: From Description to Reflection', in P. Dolan, J. Canavan and J. Pinkerton (eds.) *Family support as reflective practice,* London and Philadelphia: Jessica Kingsley Publishers, pp 280-289.

Care Council for Wales (2002) *Codes of practice for social care workers and employers of social care workers.* Cardiff: Care Council for Wales.

Care Council for Wales (2011) *National occupational standards for social work.* Cardiff: Care Council for Wales.

Carson, D. (1996) 'Risking legal repercussions', in H. Kemshall and L. Pritchard (eds) *Good practice in risk assessment and management*, vol. 1, London: Jessica Kingsley, pp 3–12.

Carter, B. (2013) 'Reflecting in groups', in C. Bulman and S. Schutz (eds) *Reflective practice in nursing* (5th edn), London: Blackwell, pp 93–120.

Cheng, I.K.S. (2010) 'Transforming practice: reflections on the use of art to develop professional knowledge and reflective practice', *Reflective Practice*, 11(4): 489–98.

Chu, W.C.K. and Tsui, M. (2008) 'The nature of practice wisdom in social work revisited', *International Social Work,* 51(1): 47-54.

Clawson, R. and Kitson, D. (2013) 'Significant incident learning process (SILP) – the experience of facilitating and evaluating the process in adult safeguarding', *Journal of Adult Protection*, 15 (5): 237–45.

Consejo General de Colegios Oficiales de Diplomados en Trabajo Social y Asistentes Sociales, Espana (1999) 'Código deontológico de la profesión de diplomado en trabajo social', ifsw.org/publications/national-codes-of-ethics/spain.

Conselho Federal de Serviço Social – CFESS (2011) 'Código de ética profissional do/a assistente social' (10ª edição), www.cfess. org.br/visualizar/menu/local/regulamentacao-da-profissao.

Cornish, S. and Preston-Shoot, M. (2013) 'Governance in adult safeguarding in Scotland since the implementation of the Adult Support and Protection (Scotland) Act 2007', *Journal of Adult Protection*, 15(5): 223–36.

Danish Association of Social Workers (2000) 'Etikvejledning: Etiske principper i socialt arbejde', ifsw.org/publications/national-codes-of-ethics/dasw-code-of-ethics/.

Darragh, E. and Taylor, B.J. (2009) 'Research and reflective practice', in P. Higham (ed.) *Post-qualifying social work: From competence to expertise*, London: Sage, pp 148–60.

de Brabandere, L. and Mikolajczak, A. (2009) *Petite philosophie de nos erreurs quotidiennes: Comment nous trompons-nous? [Philosophy of our daily small errors: How do we deceive ourselves?]*, Paris: Groupe Eyrolles.

Deaver, S.P. and McAuliffe, G. (2009) 'Reflective visual journaling during art therapy and counselling internships: a qualitative study', *Reflective Practice*, 10(5): 615–32.

Deutscher Berufsverband für Soziale Arbeit (1997) 'Berufsethische Prinzipien des DBSH', ifsw.org/publications/national-codes-of-ethics/germany/.

Devaney, J., Bunting, L., Hayes, D. and Lazenbatt, A. (2013) *Translating learning into action: An overview of learning arising from case management reviews in Northern Ireland 2003–2008*. Belfast: Queen's University Belfast, National Society for the Prevention of Cruelty to Children Northern Ireland and Department of Health, Social Services and Public Safety.

Dewey, J. (1910) *How we think*, New York, NY: D.C. Heath.

DfE (2014) *Knowledge and skills statement for child and family social work*. London: Department for Education.

DH (2015a) *Knowledge and skills statement for social workers in adult services*. London: Department of Health.

DH (2015b) *Mental Health Act 1983: Code of practice*. London: The Stationery Office.

DH (2016) *Care and support statutory guidance: Issued under the Care Act 2014*. London: Department of Health.

DHSSPS (2011) *Guidance to Safeguarding Board for Northern Ireland*. Belfast: Department of Health, Social Services and Public Safety.

Dillon, C. (2003) *Learning from mistakes in clinical practice*, Belmont, CA: Brooks/Cole.

Doel, M., Shardlow, S., Sawdon, C. and Sawdon, D. (1996) *Teaching social work practice: A programme of exercises and activities towards the practice teaching award*, Aldershot: Ashgate.

Dolan, P., Pinkerton, J. and Canavan, J. (2006) 'Family support: from description to reflection', in P. Dolan, J. Canavan and J. Pinkerton, J. (eds) *Family support as reflective practice*, London: Jessica Kingsley Publishers, pp 11–26.

Dominelli, L. (2004) *Social work: Theory and practice for a changing profession*, Cambridge: Polity.

Fincher S. and Petre, M. (eds) (2004) *Computer science education research*, New York: Taylor and Francis.

Fish, S., Munro, E. and Bairstow, S. (2009) *Learning together to safeguard children: Developing a multi-agency systems approach for case reviews*. London: Social Care Institute for Excellence.

Flanagan, J. (1954) 'The critical incident technique', *Psychological Bulletin*, 51(4): 327–58.

Flynn, M., Keywood, K. and Williams, S. (2011) 'Critical decisions and questions regarding serious case reviews: ideas from North West England', *Journal of Adult Protection*, 13 (4), 213–29.

Folkman, J.R. (2006) *The power of feedback: 35 principles for turning feedback from others into personal and professional change*, Hoboken: John Wiley & Sons.

Fook, J. and Gardner, F. (2007) *Practising critical reflection: A resource handbook*, Berkshire: McGraw-Hill Open University Press.

Fook, J., White, S. and Gardner, F. (2006) 'Critical reflection: a review of contemporary literature and understanding', in S. White, J. Fook and F. Gardner (eds) *Critical reflection in health and social care*, Berkshire: Open University Press, pp 3-20.

Forbes, W., Hudson, R. and Soufian, M. (2014) 'Thinking fast and slowly about financial decisions: Gigerenzer's critique of the Kahneman and Tversky research program', paper presented at the Twenty-first Annual Conference of the Multinational Finance Society, Praha, 29 June–1 July, pp 1–24.

Forte, J.A. (2014) *Skills for using theory in social work*, Abingdon: Routledge.

Foundation for Critical Thinking (1987) 'Defining critical thinking: critical thinking as defined by the National Council for Excellence in Critical Thinking', www.criticalthinking. org/pages/defining-critical-thinking/766.

Fronek, P., Kendall, M., Ungerer, G., Malt, J., Eugarde, E. and Geraghty, T. (2009) 'Too hot to handle: reflections on professional boundaries in practice', *Reflective Practice*, 10(2): 161–71.

Fronte, L. (2008) 'Se il fallimento è anche uno strumento di lavoro' [If failure is also a working tool], *Animazione Sociale*, 38(3): 69–77.

Frost, L. (2016) 'Exploring the concepts of recognition and shame for social work', *Journal of Social Work Practice*, online, pp. 1–16.

Frost, S. (2006) 'Recasting individual practice through reflection on narratives', in S. White, J. Fook and F. Gardner (eds) *Critical reflection in health and social care*, Berkshire: Open University Press, pp 107–17.

Gelb, M.J. (1996) *Thinking for a change: Discovering the power to create, communicate, and lead*, New York: Harmony Books.

Ghaye, A. and Ghaye, K. (1998) *Teaching and learning through critical reflective practice*, London: David Fulton.

Ghaye, T. (2008) *Building the reflective healthcare organisation*, Oxford: Blackwell.

Gherardi, S. (1989) *Sociologia delle decisioni organizzative [Sociology of organisational decisions]*, Bologna: Il Mulino.

Gibbs, G. (1988) *Learning by doing: A guide to teaching and learning methods,* London: Further Education Unit.

Gigerenzer, G. (2007) *Gut feelings: The intelligence of the unconscious*, London: Penguin.

Gigerenzer, G., Todd, P. M. and the ABC Research Group (eds) (1999) *Simple heuristics that make us smart*, New York: Oxford University Press.

Goleman, D. (1995) *Emotional Intelligence: Why it can matter more than IQ*, New York: Bantam Books.

Goodman, J. (1984) 'Reflection and teacher education: a case study and theoretical analysis', *Interchange: A Quarterly Review of Education*, 15(3): 9–26.

Gould, N. (1996) 'Using imagery in reflective learning', in N. Gould and I. Taylor (eds), *Reflective learning for social work*, Aldershot: Ashgate, pp 63–77.

Gould, N. (2004) 'Introduction: The learning organization and reflective practice – the emergence of a concept', in N. Gould and M. Baldwin (eds), *Social work, critical reflection and the learning organization*, Aldershot: Ashgate, pp 1–9.

Gould, N. and Baldwin, M. (eds) (2004) *Social work, critical reflection and the learning organization*, Aldershot: Ashgate.

Green Lister, P. (2012) *Integrating social work theory and practice: A practical skills guide*, London: Routledge.

Green Lister, P. and Crisp, B. (2007) 'Critical incident analyses: a practice learning tool for students and practitioners', *Practice*, 19(1): 47–60.

Habermas, J. (1971) *Knowledge and human interests*, Boston, MA: Beacon Press.

Habermas, J. (1984) *Theory of communicative action*, Boston, MA: Beacon Press.

Harford, T. (2011) *Adapt: Why success always starts with failure*, London: Little Brown.

Harris, J. (2014) '(Against) Neoliberal social work', *Critical and Radical Social Work*, 2(1): 7–22.

Hathaway, P. (1990) *Giving and receiving criticism: Your key to interpersonal success. Practical guidelines for better life management*, Los Altos: Crisp Publications.

HCPC (2012a) *Standards of proficiency: Social workers in England*. London: Health & Care Professions Council.

HCPC (2012b) *Standards of conduct, performance and ethics*. London: Health & Care Professions Council.

Hettrich, C.M., Mather, R.C., Sethi, M.K., Nunley, R.M., Jahangir, A.A. and the Washington Health Policy Fellows (2010) 'The costs of defensive medicine', *AAOS Now*, December: 8–10.

HM Government (2015) *Working together to safeguard children: A guide to inter-agency working to safeguard and promote the welfare of children*, London: The Stationery Office.

Holly, M.L. (1988) 'Reflective writing and the spirit of enquiry', *Cambridge Journal of Education*, 19(1): 71–80.

Home Office (2013) *Multi-agency statutory guidance for the conduct of domestic homicide reviews*, London: The Stationery Office.

IASSW and IFSW (2004) 'Ethics in Social Work, Statement of Principles', ifsw.org/policies/statement-of-ethical-principles/.

IFSW (International Federation of Social Workers) (2004) 'Ethics in social work: statement of principles', Geneva, Switzerland: International Federation of Social Workers (IFSW), ifsw.org/policies/statement-of-ethical-principles/.

IFSW (International Federation of Social Workers) and IASSW (International Association of School of Social Work) (2014) 'Global definition of social work', ifsw.org/get-involved/global-definition-of-social-work/.

IFSW (International Federation of Social Workers) (2016) 'National codes of ethics', http://ifsw.org/publications/national-codes-of-ethics/.

Ingram, R., Fenton, J., Hodson, A. and Jindal-Snape, D. (2014) *Reflective social work practice*, Basingstoke: Palgrave.

Isaac, S. and Michael, W.B. (1989) *Handbook in research and evaluation for education and the behavioural sciences*, San Diego: EdiTS Publisher.

Japanese Association of Certified Social Workers (2004) 'Code of ethics of social worker', https://www.jacsw.or.jp/06_kokusai/IFSW/files/06_koryo_e.html.

Jasper, M. (2003) *Beginning reflective practice,* Cheltenham: Nelson Thornes.

Jasper, M. (2004) 'Using journals and diaries within reflective practice' in C. Bulman and S. Schutz (eds) *Reflective practice in nursing* (3rd edn), London: Blackwell, pp 94–112.

Jefferson, M. (2016) *Mistakes greatest quotes: Quick, short, medium or long quotes. Find the perfect mistakes quotations for all occasions: Spicing up letters, speeches, and everyday conversations*, n.a.: Emereo.

Johnson, L.A. (2003) *A toolbox for humanity: 3000 years of thought*, Victoria: Trafford.

Jones, S. (2013) *Critical learning for social work students*, London: Learning Matters.

Kadushin, A. and Kadushin, G. (2013) *The social work interview* (5th edn), New York, Columbia University Press.

Kahneman, N. (2002) 'Maps of bounded rationality: a perspective on intuitive judgment and choice', Nobel Price Lecture, nobelprize.org/economics/laureates/2002/kahnemann-lecture.pdf.

Kahneman, N. (2011) *Thinking, fast and slow*, London: Allen Lane.

Kaplan–Williams, S. (1980) *The Jungian-Senoi dreamwork manual*, Berkeley, CA: Journey Press.

Kemshall, H. (2001) *Risk assessment and management of known sexual and violent offenders: A review of current issues*, London: Crown.

Kinsella, E.A. (2010) 'The art of reflective practice in health and social care: reflections on the legacy of Donald Schön', *Reflective Practice*, 11(4): 565–75.

Knott, C. and Scragg, T. (2013) *Reflective practice in social work* (3rd edn), London: Sage.

Knott, C. and Spafford, J. (2013) 'Getting started', in C. Knott and T. Scragg (eds) *Reflective practice in social work* (3rd edn), London: Sage, pp 16–33.

Kogerus, M. and Tschäppeler, R. (2011) *The decision book: Fifty models for stategic thinking*, London: Profile Books.

Kolb, D.A. (1984) *Experiential learning: Experience as the source of learning and development*, Englewood Cliffs, NJ: Prentice Hall.

LGA (2014) *The standards for employers of social workers in England*. London: Local Government Association.

Lia, P. (2014) 'Using Gibbs' reflective cycle', Learning Support Tutor, Disability Advisory Service, King's College London, https://www.kcl.ac.uk/campuslife/services/disability/online resources/Using-Gibbs-Reflective-Cycle-in-Coursework.pdf.

Maclean, S. (2010) *The social work pocket guide to reflective practice*, Whitby: De Sitter.

McCray, J. (2013) 'Reflective practice for collaborative working', in C. Knott and T. Scragg (2013) *Reflective practice in social work* (3rd edn), London: Sage, pp 144–55.

McIntosh, P. (2010) *Action research and reflective practice: Creative and visual methods to facilitate reflection and learning. Understanding educational research,* Abingdon: Routledge.

McLaughlin, H. (2009) 'What's in a name: "client", "patient", "customer", "expert by experience", "service user": what's next?', *British Journal of Social Work*, 39(6): 1101–17

Manthorpe, J. and Martineau, S. (2015) 'What can and cannot be learned from serious case reviews of the care and treatment of adults with learning disabilities in England? Messages for social workers', *British Journal of Social Work*, 45(1): 331–48.

Merton, R. and Barber, E. (2004) *The travels and adventures of serendipity: A study in sociological semantics and the sociology of science,* Princeton, NJ: Princeton University Press.

Merton, R.K. (1948) 'The self-fulfilling prophecy', *Antioch Review*, 8(2): 193–210.

Mezirow, J. (1981) 'A critical theory of adult learning and education', *Adult Education*, 32(1): 3–24.

Moon, J. (2006) *Learning journals: A handbook for reflective practice and professional development* (2nd edn), Abingdon: Routledge.

Motterlini, M. (2006a) *Economia emotiva: Cosa si nasconde dietro I nostri conti quotidiani [Emotional economy: What lies behind our daily accounts],* Milano: Rizzoli.

Motterlini, M. (2006b) 'Scommesse incoerenti' [Inconsistent betting], *Sole 24 Ore,* 3 Sept.: 34.

Motterlini, M. and Crupi, V. (2006) 'Errori e decisioni in medicina' [Errors and decisions in medicine], in V. Crupi, G.F. Gensini and M. Motterlini (eds) *La dimensione cognitiva dell'errore in medicina [The cognitive dimension of error in medicine],* Milano: FrancoAngeli, pp 11–42.

Munro, E. (1996) 'Avoidable and unavoidable mistakes in child protection work', *British Journal of Social Work*, 26(6): 793–808.

Munro, E. (2011) *The Munro review of child protection, final report: A child-centred system,* London: The Stationery Office.

National Association of Social Workers (USA) (2008) 'Code of ethics', www.socialworkers.org/pubs/code/code.asp.

Northern Ireland Social Care Council (2002) *Codes of practice for social care workers and employers of social care workers.* Belfast: Northern Ireland Social Care Council.

Northern Ireland Social Care Council (2011) *National occupational standards for social work.* Belfast: Northern Ireland Social Care Council.

Ordine Assistenti Sociali – National Council (2009) 'Code of ethics for social workers', Rome, www.cnoas.info/files/000000/00000018.pdf.

Parry, I. (2014) 'Adult serious case reviews: lessons for housing providers', *Journal of Social Welfare and Family Law,* 36(2): 168–89.

Penn, K. and Sastry, A. (2014) *Fail better: Design smart mistakes and succeed sooner,* Boston, MA: Harvard Business Review Press.

Perrow, C. (2001) 'Accidents, normal', in N.J. Smelser and P.B. Baltes (eds) *International encyclopedia of the social and behavioral sciences,* vol. 1, Amsterdam: Elsevier, pp 33–8.

Polanyi, M. (1966) *The tacit dimension,* Chicago: University of Chicago Press.

Preston-Shoot, M. (2014) *Making good decisions: Law for social work practice.* Basingstoke: Palgrave Macmillan.

Ravasi, G. (1996) 'The master in the Bible', Acts of the International Seminar on 'Jesus, the Master', Ariccia, 14–24 October, www.stpauls.it/studi/maestro/inglese/ravasi/ingrav02.htm.

Rawal, S. (2009) '… as I engaged in reflection: a play in three acts', *Reflective Practice,* 10(1): 27–32.

Reason, J. (1990) *Human error,* Cambridge: Cambridge University Press.

Reason, J. (2000) 'Human error: models and management', *British Medical Journal,* 320(7237): 768–70.

Reber, A., Reber, E. and Allen, R. (2009) *Dictionary of psychology* (4th edn), London: Penguin.

Redmond, B. (2004) *Reflection in action: Developing reflective practice in health and social services,* Aldershot: Ashgate.

Rilke, R. (1945) *Letters to a young poet,* London: Sidgwick and Jackson.

Rogers, C. (1969) *Freedom to learn: A view of what education might become* (1st edn), Columbus, OH: Charles E. Merill.

Rolfe, G., Freshwater, D. and Jasper, M. (2001) *Critical reflection for nursing and the helping professions: A users guide*, Basingstoke: Palgrave.

Ruch, G. (2009) *Post-qualifying child care social work: Developing reflective practice*, London: Sage.

Russell, J.A. (1980) 'A circumplex model of affect', *Journal of Personality and Social Psychology*, 6(39): 1161–78.

Schön, D.A. (1983) *The reflective practitioner: How professionals think in action*, New York: Basic Books.

Schön, D. A. (1987) *Educating the reflective practitioner: Toward a new design for teaching and learning in the professions*, San Francisco: Jossey-Bass.

Schulz, K. (2010) *Being wrong: Adventures in the margin of error*, New York: HarperCollins.

Scottish Social Services Council (2009) *Codes of Practice for Social Services Workers and Employers*, Dundee: Scottish Social Services Council.

Scottish Social Services Council (2011) *National Occupational Standards for Social Work,* Dundee: Scottish Social Services Council.

Seneca, L. (1979) *Letters from a stoic: Epistulae morales ad Lucilium*, Harmondsworth: Penguin Books.

Shafir, E. (1993) 'Choosing versus rejecting: why some options are both better and worse than others', *Memory & Cognition*, 21: 546–56.

Sicora, A. (2010) *Errore e apprendimento nelle professioni di aiuto: Fare più errori per fare meno danni? [Error and learning in the helping professions: Make more mistakes to do less damage?]*, Santarcangelo di Romagna (RN): Maggioli.

Sicora, A. (2013) *La violenza contro gli operatori dei servizi sociali e sanitari [Violence against workers in health and social services],* Roma: Carocci.

Sicora, A. (2014) 'Aggression towards helping professions: violence as communication, listening as prevention?' *Argumentum*, 6(2): 154–65.

Singapore Association of Social Workers (2004) 'SASW code of professional ethics', Singapore, www.fas.nus.edu.sg/swk/doc/gdsw_2013/Appendix_J_SASW_Code_of_ethics.pdf.

Smith, M.J. (1975) *Not one word has been omitted: When I say no, I feel guilty*, New York: Bentam.

Snyder, S. (2003) 'How to ask a smart question', faculty.gvc.edu/ssnyder/121/Goodquestions.html.

Social Workers Registration Board, Kahui Whakamana Tauwhiro (2014) 'Code of conduct for social workers', http://www.swrb.govt.nz/doc-man/code-of-conduct-1/323-code-of-conduct

South African Council for Social Service Professions (2007) 'Policy guidelines for course of conduct, code of ethics and the rules for social workers', www.sacssp.co.za/Content/documents/EthicsCode.pdf.

Sparrow, J. (2009) 'Impact of emotions associated with reflecting upon the past', *Reflective Practice*, 10(5): 567–576.

Stimson, W.R. (2009) 'Using dreams to train the reflective practitioner: the Ullman dream group in social work education', *Reflective Practice*, 10(5): 577–87.

Stroobants, H. (2009) 'On humour and reflection', *Reflective Practice*, 10(1): 5–12.

Swedish Association of Graduates in Social Science, Personnel and Public Administration, Economics and Social Work (2008) 'Ethics in social work: an ethical code for social work professionals', Akademikerförbundet SSR, Stockholm, cdn.ifsw.org/assets/Socialt_arbete_etik_08_Engelsk_LR.pdf.

Tate, S. (2013) 'Writing to learn: writing reflectively?, in C. Bulman and S. Schutz (eds) *Reflective practice in nursing* (5th edn), London: Blackwell, pp 53–92.

Tavris, G. and Aronson, E. (2007) *Mistakes were made (but not by me)*, New York: Harcourt.

Taylor, B.J. (2010) *Reflective practice for healthcare professionals* (3rd edn), Berkshire: McGraw-Hill.

Taylor, B.J. (2013) *Professional decision making and risk in social work* (2nd edn), London: Sage.

Taylor, C. (2006) 'Practising reflexivity: narrative, reflection and the moral order', in S. White, J. Fook and F. Gardner (eds) *Critical reflection in health and social care*, Berkshire: Open University Press, pp 73–88.

Thomas, J. (2004) 'Using "critical incident analysis" to promote critical reflection and holistic assessment", in N. Gould and M. Baldwin (eds) *Social work, critical reflection and the learning organization*, Aldershot: Ashgate, pp 101–15.

Thompson, N. (2010) *Theorizing social work practice*, New York: Palgrave Macmillan.

Thompson, S. and Thompson, N. (2008) *The critically reflective practitioner*, New York: Palgrave Macmillan.

Tokolahi, E. (2010) 'Case study: development of a drawing⊠ based journal to facilitate reflective inquiry', *Reflective Practice*, 11(2): 157–70.

Tugend, A. (2011) *Better by mistake: The unexpected benefits of being wrong*, London: Riverhead Books.

Union of Social Educators and Social Workers (2003) 'The ethical guideline of social educator and social worker', Moscow, cdn.ifsw.org/assets/Russian_ethical.pdf.

Union of Social Workers (2007) 'Code of professional ethics of the social workers In Israel', Tel Aviv, ifsw.org/publications/national-codes-of-ethics/israel/.

Vincent, S. and Petch, A. (2012) *Audit and analysis of significant case reviews*. Edinburgh: Scottish Government.

Vitullo, A. (2006) *Leadership riflessive: la ricerca di anima nelle organizzazioni [Reflective leadership: Soul-searching in organizations]*, Milano: Apogeo.

Watzlawick, P. (1983) *The situation is hopeless, but not serious (the pursuit of unhappiness)*, New York: Norton.

Watzlawick, P., Beaving, J. and Jackson, D. (1967) *Pragmatic of human communication,* New York: Norton.

White, S., Fook, J. and Gardner, F. (eds.) (2006) *Critical reflection in health and social care*, Berkshire: Open University Press.

Wormeli, R. (2003) *Day one and beyond: Practical matters for new middle-level teachers*, Portland: Stenhouse Publishers.

Index

Printed and bound by CPI Group (UK) Ltd, Croydon, CR0 4YY

31/07/2024

14535085-0003